STUDY GUIDE TO

The American Psychiatric Press
Textbook of Geriatric Psychiatry,
Second Edition

STUDY GUIDE TO

The American Psychiatric Press Textbook of Geriatric Psychiatry, Second Edition

F. M. Baker, M.D., M.P.H.

Professor, Department of Psychiatry
University of Maryland School of Medicine
Medical Director, Lower Shore Clinic
Salisbury, Maryland

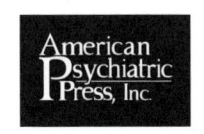

American Psychiatric Press, Inc.

Washington, DC
London, England

Note: The authors have worked to ensure that all information in this book concerning drug dosages, schedules, and routes of administration is accurate as of the time of publication and consistent with standards set by the U.S. Food and Drug Administration and the general medical community. As medical research and practice advance, however, therapeutic standards may change. For this reason and because human and mechanical errors sometimes occur, we recommend that readers follow the advice of a physician who is directly involved in their care or the care of a member of their family. A product's current package insert should be consulted for full prescribing and safety information.

Books published by the American Psychiatric Press, Inc., represent the views and opinions of the individual authors and do not necessarily represent the policies and opinions of the Press or the American Psychiatric Association.

Copyright © 2001 American Psychiatric Press, Inc.
ALL RIGHTS RESERVED
Manufactured in the United States of America on acid-free paper

04 03 02 01   4 3 2 1
First Edition

American Psychiatric Press, Inc.
1400 K Street, N.W.
Washington, DC 20005
www.appi.org

This book is dedicated to my parents, Alzora Baker and Joseph L. Baker, C.S., and my godparents, Fannie G. Ford and David Ford Jr. Their love, interest, and encouragement remain the foundation of my achievements.

Contents

Preface ix

SECTION I

The Basic Science of Geriatric Psychiatry

CHAPTER 1   The Myth, History, and Science of Aging. 3

CHAPTER 2   Physiological and Clinical Considerations of the Geriatric Patient. 7

CHAPTER 3   Perceptual Changes With Aging 11

CHAPTER 4   Neuroanatomy and Neuropathology of Aging. 15

CHAPTER 5   Chemical Messengers. 17

CHAPTER 6   Genetics and Geriatric Psychiatry 21

CHAPTER 7   Psychological Aspects of Normal Aging 25

CHAPTER 8   Social and Economic Factors Related to Psychiatric Disorders in Late Life. 31

CHAPTER 9   Epidemiology of Psychiatric Disorders in Late Life . . . 35

SECTION II

The Diagnostic Interview in Late Life

CHAPTER 10   The Psychiatric Interview of the Geriatric Patient. . . . 43

CHAPTER 11   Use of the Laboratory in the Diagnostic Workup of Older Adults 49

Section III

Psychiatric Disorders in Late Life

CHAPTER 12	Cognitive Disorders	59
CHAPTER 13	Mood Disorders	65
CHAPTER 14	Schizophrenia and Paranoid Disorders	79
CHAPTER 15	Anxiety and Panic Disorders	85
CHAPTER 16	Somatoform and Psychosexual Disorders	89
CHAPTER 17	Bereavement and Adjustment Disorders	105
CHAPTER 18	Sleep and Chronobiological Disturbances	111
CHAPTER 19	Alcohol and Drug Problems	121

Section IV

Treatment of Psychiatric Disorders in Late Life

CHAPTER 20	Pharmacological Treatment	133
CHAPTER 21	Diet, Nutrition, and Exercise	149
CHAPTER 22	Psychotherapy	155
CHAPTER 23	Clinical Psychiatry in the Nursing Home	169
CHAPTER 24	The Continuum of Care: Movement Toward the Community	179

Preface

The purpose of the *Study Guide to The American Psychiatric Press Textbook of Geriatric Psychiatry, Second Edition,* is to provide readers of *The American Psychiatric Press Textbook of Geriatric Psychiatry,* Second Edition, with an opportunity to evaluate their understanding of the material contained in that text (the complete table of contents to the textbook follows this preface). The textbook is a one-volume, comprehensive, clinically focused, up-to-date textbook that reviews the field of geriatric psychiatry. Its contents provide the crucial knowledge that medical students, psychiatric residents, psychiatrists, geriatric psychiatry fellows, geriatric medicine, and primary care physicians with a special interest in geriatric psychiatry may require in order to provide high-quality care to the older patient and his or her family. The study guide was developed for students, residents, fellows, and clinicians to assess their knowledge of the important basic science foundations, diagnostic issues, psychiatric disorders in late life, psychiatric treatments, and special sites of treatment in the field of geriatric psychiatry.

The American Psychiatric Press Textbook of Geriatric Psychiatry, Second Edition, was written with the expectation that readers would not necessarily choose to read the entire book from Chapter 1 to the end. Consequently, the questions have been designed so that readers, who may read only specific chapters in any one of the four sections of the book, can receive an appropriate evaluation of their knowledge of each of these particular areas. In addition, because there is an increasing emphasis on continuing medical education and assessment of one's knowledge base through state licensing boards and national certifying boards, use of the study guide should provide valuable assistance to readers to ensure that their understanding of many important areas in geriatric psychiatry is satisfactory.

In summary, I hope that you will find the *Study Guide to The American Psychiatric Press Textbook of Geriatric Psychiatry, Second Edition,* to be a useful addition to your continuing medical education needs. Your comments and critiques of the study guide are welcomed so that it may be improved and streamlined for the next edition.

Acknowledgments

The support and collaboration of my colleagues and mentors must be acknowledged. Without the clinical skills and research activities of practicing geriatric psychiatrists, this study guide would not have been possible.

The dedication and perseverance of the administrative staff of the Department of Psychiatry of the Indiana University School of Medicine contributed to the preparation of this manuscript. A special acknowledgment is made to Francine L. Bray who brought this project to closure.

THE AMERICAN PSYCHIATRIC PRESS
TEXTBOOK OF GERIATRIC PSYCHIATRY

Second Edition

Edited by
Ewald W. Busse, M.D., and Dan G. Blazer, M.D., Ph.D.

Contents

Preface
Ewald W. Busse, M.D., and Dan G. Blazer, M.D., Ph.D.

The Basic Science of Geriatric Psychiatry

1. The Myth, History, and Science of Aging
   Ewald W. Busse, M.D.
2. Physiological and Clinical Considerations of the Geriatric Patient
   John W. Rowe, M.D., and Cathryn A. J. Devons, M.D., M.P.H.
3. Perceptual Changes With Aging
   Gail R. Marsh, Ph.D.
4. Neuroanatomy and Neuropathology of Aging
   F. Stephen Vogel, M.D.
5. Chemical Messengers
   Garth Bissette, Ph.D.
6. Genetics and Geriatric Psychiatry
   Ewald W. Busse, M.D., and Dan G. Blazer, M.D., Ph.D.
7. Psychological Aspects of Normal Aging
   Ilene C. Siegler, Ph.D., M.P.H., Leonard W. Poon, Ph.D., David J. Madden, Ph.D., and Kathleen A. Welsh, Ph.D.
8. Social and Economic Factors Related to Psychiatric Disorders in Late Life
   Linda K. George, Ph.D.
9. Epidemiology of Psychiatric Disorders in Late Life
   Dan G. Blazer, M.D., Ph.D.

The Diagnostic Interview in Late Life

10. The Psychiatric Interview of the Geriatric Patient
    Dan G. Blazer, M.D., Ph.D.

11 Use of the Laboratory in the Diagnostic Workup of Older Adults
    Dan G. Blazer, M.D., Ph.D., Ewald W. Busse, M.D.,
    W. Edward Craighead, Ph.D., and Donald D. Evans, Ph.D.

Psychiatric Disorders in Late Life

12 Cognitive Disorders
    Elaine R. Peskind, M.D., and Murray A. Raskind, M.D.

13 Mood Disorders
    Dan G. Blazer, M.D., Ph.D., and Harold G. Koenig, M.D., M.H.Sc.

14 Schizophrenia and Paranoid Disorders
    Harold G. Koenig, M.D., M.H.Sc., Caron Christison, M.D.,
    George Christison, M.D., and Dan G. Blazer, M.D., Ph.D.

15 Anxiety and Panic Disorders
    Javaid I. Sheikh, M.D.

16 Somatoform and Psychosexual Disorders
    Ewald W. Busse, M.D.

17 Bereavement and Adjustment Disorders
    Dolores Gallagher-Thompson, Ph.D., and Larry W. Thompson, Ph.D.

18 Sleep and Chronobiological Disturbances
    Thomas C. Neylan, M.D., Mary G. De May, M.D., and
    Charles F. Reynolds III, M.D.

19 Alcohol and Drug Problems
    Dan G. Blazer, M.D., Ph.D.

Treatment of Psychiatric Disorders in Late Life

20 Pharmacological Treatment
    Jonathan Davidson, M.D.

21 Diet, Nutrition, and Exercise
    Robert J. Sullivan Jr., M.D.

22 Psychotherapy
    Keith G. Meador, M.D., M.P.H., and Claudia D. Davis, R.N., M.S.N.

23 Clinical Psychiatry in the Nursing Home
    Joel E. Streim, M.D., and Ira R. Katz, M.D., Ph.D.

24 The Continuum of Care: Movement Toward the Community
    George L. Maddox, Ph.D., Karen Steinhauser, M.A., and
    Elise Bolda, M.S.P.H., Ph.D.

25 The Past and Future of Geriatric Psychiatry
    Ewald W. Busse, M.D., and Dan G. Blazer. M.D., Ph.D.

Section I

The Basic Science of Geriatric Psychiatry

Chapter 1

The Myth, History, and Science of Aging

QUESTIONS

Directions: **Select the single best response for each of the following questions:**

1.1 The best general definition of aging is
   A. The adverse effects of the passage of time.
   B. The physical changes that develop in adulthood resulting in a decline in efficiency of function and terminating in death.
   C. Changes in appearance and ability.
   D. All of these.
   E. None of these.

1.2 The stochastic theory of aging, as developed by atomic scientist Leo Szilard,
   A. Required a hit.
   B. Required the presence of a fault (a congenital absence or impairment) of a region of a gene essential to cell function.
   C. Required both a hit and the presence of a fault that, when combined, increased the risk of a random outcome of impaired cell function or cell death.
   D. All of these.
   E. None of these.

1.3 The belief that older men can absorb vitality and youth from sex and intimacy with a woman, particularly a younger woman, is termed
   A. *Hyperborean legend*.
   B. *The fountain of youth*.
   C. *Gerocomy*.
   D. All of these.
   E. None of these.

1.4 Changes in the normal linkage of collagen molecules or between glucose and protein have been presented as biologic causes of aging. These theories of aging are termed

   A. *Eversion theory* and *glycosylation theory*.
   B. *Hyperborean theory* and *glycosylation theory*.
   C. *Glycosylation theory* and *hyperborean theory*.
   D. *Eversion theory*.
   E. None of these.

Directions: **For each of the statements below, one or more of the answers is correct. Choose**

   A. If 1, 2, and 3 are correct.
   B. If only 1 and 3 are correct.
   C. If only 2 and 4 are correct.
   D. If only 4 is correct.
   E. If all are correct.

1.5 The components of the process of aging have been separated into
   1. Primary aging.
   2. Acquired decremental aging.
   3. Secondary aging.
   4. Hereditary aging.

1.6 Descriptive changes associated with aging include
   1. Dry wrinkles.
   2. Seborrheic skin and gray hair.
   3. Decayed teeth and decreased height.
   4. Increased abdominal girth.

1.7 Markers of chronological age include
   1. Changes in appearance.
   2. The ability to perform activities of daily living.
   3. The ability to work.
   4. The absence of change in metabolic dimensions.

1.8 A nonenzymatic reaction between glucose and protein is termed
   1. *Glycosylation.*
   2. *Browning reaction.*
   3. *Maillard reaction.*
   4. *Cerami reaction.*

1.9 The Greek legend of the Hyperboreans described a group of people
   1. Who lived in the east.
   2. Lived in perpetual summer.
   3. Died at the age of 30.
   4. Who were free of all natural ills.

ANSWERS

1.1 The answer is **B**. The physical changes that develop in adulthood resulting in a decline in efficiency of function and terminating in death **(p. 11)** is the best general definition of aging.

1.2 The answer is **C**. The stochastic theory of aging—as developed by atomic scientist Leo Szilard—required both a hit and the presence of a fault that, when combined, increased the risk of a random outcome of impaired cell function or cell death. Szilard defined a *hit* as any event that could alter a chromosome **(p. 14)**. He believed that all organisms carried a load of faults. Szilard defined a fault as the congenital absence or impairment of one of the genes essential to cell function **(p. 14)**.

1.3 The answer is **C**. The belief that older men can absorb vitality and youth from sex and intimacy with a woman, particularly a younger woman, is termed *gerocomy* **(p. 4)**.

1.4 The answer is **A**. The eversion theory of aging relates age-related change to a change in the ester bonding within the collagen molecule. With aging, ester linkages bind together individual collagen molecules changing the characteristics of connective tissue. Glycosylation may also cause this cross linkage **(p. 15)**.

1.5 The answer is **B**. The process of aging has been separated into two components. *Primary aging* describes the intrinsic, hereditary factors of the organism. *Secondary aging* refers to defects and disabilities caused by environmental factors or trauma **(pp. 11–12)**.

1.6 The answer is **E**. The dry wrinkles, seborrheic skin, gray hair, decayed teeth, decreased height, and increased abdominal girth provide a descriptive picture of many elder persons **(p. 12)**.

1.7 The answer is **A**. Changes in appearance and the ability to perform tasks associated with activities of daily living and working have been used as markers of chronological age. The age-related metabolic changes affect drug absorption, distribution, destruction, excretion, pharmacokinetics, and drug binding **(p. 12)**.

1.8 The answer is **A**. A nonenzymatic reaction between glucose and protein is termed *glycosylation* and is also called the *browning reaction* or the *Maillard reaction*. By this nonenzymatic process, glucose is added randomly to any of several sites along the peptide chain. Many of the products of glycosylation can link with adjacent proteins **(p. 15)**. Diabetic studies provided evidence that glycosylation could potentially damage the body by forming irreversible cross links between adjacent protein molecules **(p. 15)**.

1.9 The answer is **D**. The Greek legend of the Hyperboreans described a group of people who lived beyond the north wind in a region of perpetual sunshine, free from all natural ills. Living to an extreme old age, they ended their sated lives by jumping into the sea **(p. 4)**.

CHAPTER 2

Physiological and Clinical Considerations of the Geriatric Patient

QUESTIONS

Directions: **Select the single best response for each of the following questions:**

2.1 The increased levels of insulin in the elderly are associated with
- A. Decreased levels of triglycerides.
- B. Increased levels of high-density lipoprotein cholesterol.
- C. Decreased levels of high-density lipoprotein cholesterol.
- D. All of these.
- E. None of these.

2.2 A normal consequence of aging that has direct clinical effects is
- A. Changing glucose tolerance.
- B. Menopause.
- C. Esophageal changes.
- D. All of these.
- E. None of these.

2.3 The physiological changes of normal aging in the absence of disease are very
- A. Consistent.
- B. Variable.
- C. Discrete.
- D. All of these.
- E. None of these.

2.4 A significant predictor of future mortality among community-resident elderly was

A. Hematocrit.
B. Thyroid function.
C. Forced vital capacity.
D. All of these.
E. None of these

Directions: **For each of the statements below, one or more of the answers is correct. Choose**

A. If 1, 2, and 3 are correct.
B. If only 1 and 3 are correct.
C. If only 2 and 4 are correct.
D. If only 4 is correct.
E. If all are correct.

2.5 Age-related changes of clinical significance are *not* seen in

1. Parathyroid function.
2. Thyroid function.
3. Peristalsis of the esophagus.
4. The hematocrit.

2.6 Menopause has been associated with an increased risk for

1. Diabetes.
2. Osteoporosis.
3. Anemia of old age.
4. Atherosclerosis.

2.7 Physiologic changes of aging are modified by

1. Diet.
2. Exercise.
3. Environmental exposure.
4. Body composition.

2.8 Age changes that have direct clinical effects include

1. Menopause.
2. Cataract formation.
3. Arteriosclerosis.
4. Body mass index.

2.9 Postprandial hyperinsulinemia
1. Decreases the incidence of coronary artery disease.
2. Increases the levels of triglycerides.
3. Decreases the level of high-density lipoproteins.
4. Increases the incidence of coronary artery disease.

2.10 The prevalence of systolic hypertension in the elderly is due to
1. Increased thickening of blood vessel walls.
2. Decreased compliance in the blood vessel walls.
3. Increased stiffening of the blood vessel walls.
4. Increased incidence of diabetes mellitus.

ANSWERS

2.1 The answer is **C**. The increased levels of insulin in the elderly are associated with *increased* levels of triglycerides and *decreased* levels of high-density lipoprotein cholesterol, which increase the risk for heart disease **(p. 31)**.

2.2 The answer is **B**. Although a normal change of aging, menopause increases the risk of osteoporosis and atherosclerosis **(p. 29)**.

2.3 The answer is **B**. In many cases, the physiologic changes occurring with normal aging are very variable **(p. 26)** and associated with attributable risk factors for the development of illnesses that are potentially modifiable.

2.4 The answer is **C**. Longitudinal studies have found that forced vital capacity is a statistically significant predictor of mortality among community-resident elderly **(p. 40)**.

2.5 The answer is **E**. In the absence of disease, the development of a very mild form of hyperparathyroidism in the elderly is due to a decrease in renal mass **(p. 31)** and is not a major contributor to the development of osteoporosis **(p. 32)**. Aging has no significant effect on thyroid gland function or on the results of diagnostic thyroid function tests **(p. 32)**. Without disease, the modest decrease in the amplitude of esophageal peristalsis is not clinically significant **(p. 40)**. Data from the Framingham study found no age-related change in hematocrit among healthy community-dwelling elderly, eliminating the concept of "anemia of old age" **(p. 27)**.

2.6 The answer is **C**. An increased risk for *osteoporosis* and *atherosclerosis* has been found to be associated with menopause **(p. 29)**. The decline in circulating levels of estrogen with menopause can increase the rate of subsequent bone loss in women with low bone density. Estrogen replacement therapy at the time of menopause can aid these women and decrease the risk of fractures **(p. 34)**. Atherosclerosis is the development of plaques in the intima of the vessel that narrow the lumen of the vessel **(p. 29)**.

2.7 The answer is **E**. Recent longitudinal studies of carefully selected populations that excluded individuals with subclinical illness **(p. 25)** have shown that the observed changes in the aged may be substantially less than previously recognized. Factors such as personal habits, diet, exercise, nutrition, environmental exposures, and body composition were found to play an important role **(p. 26)**.

2.8 The answer is **A**. Three normal consequences of aging that have direct clinical effects include *menopause, cataract formation,* and *arteriosclerosis.* Increased lens opacification (cataract formation) due to posttranslational modification of central lens proteins produce increasing opacity of the lens, decreasing its ability to accommodate to near vision **(p. 29)**. Arteriosclerosis is defined as the thickening of the walls of the major arteries resulting in decreased compliance and an increased stiffening of vessels that produces an increase in systolic blood pressure, a major contributor to the prevalence of systolic hypertension in the elderly **(p. 29)**.

2.9 The answer is **D**. Postprandial hyperinsulinemia *increases* the incidence of coronary artery disease **(p. 31)**. Increased levels of insulin have been shown to be a significant and independent contributor to the incidence of coronary artery disease **(p. 31)**.

2.10 The answer is **A**. *Arteriosclerosis* is defined as the thickening of the walls of the major arteries resulting in decreased compliance and an increased stiffening of vessels that produce an increase in systolic blood pressure and is a major contributor to the prevalence of systolic hypertension in the elderly **(p. 29)**.

Chapter 3

Perceptual Changes With Aging

QUESTIONS

Directions: Select the single best response for each of the following questions:

3.1 Which of the following is false?
   A. With advanced age, the most common visual problems include cataracts, glaucoma, and macular degeneration.
   B. Near vision begins to noticeably decrease between the ages of 40–55.
   C. Contrast sensitivity uses the Snellen chart to determine acuity for distant objects.
   D. All of the above.
   E. None of the above.

3.2 Visual changes experienced by the elderly include
   A. Decrease in the ability to identify a detailed target.
   B. Lower flicker fusion threshold.
   C. A decline in peripheral vision of 67% by age 75.
   D. All of the above.
   E. None of the above.

3.3 Sensory changes experienced by the elderly include
   A. Decrease in hearing high-frequency sounds.
   B. A decline in peripheral vision.
   C. A decreased ability to distinguish blue-green hues.
   D. All of the above.
   E. None of the above.

12   Study Guide to the Textbook of Geriatric Psychiatry, Second Edition

Directions: **For each of the statements below, one or more of the answers is correct. Choose**

   A. If 1, 2, and 3 are correct.
   B. If only 1 and 3 are correct.
   C. If only 2 and 4 are correct.
   D. If only 4 is correct.
   E. If all are correct.

3.4   The components of taste perception include
   1. Salty.
   2. Sweet.
   3. Sour.
   4. Bitter.

3.5   Factors contributing to the decreased sensitivity of the chochlea to sound include
   1. Loss of elasticity of the basilar membrane.
   2. Loss of sensory receptors on basilar membrane.
   3. Loss of neurons in the eighth cranial nerve.
   4. Atrophy of the stria vascularis.

ANSWERS

3.1   The answer is **C.** Contrast sensitivity is another method of testing acuity **(p. 51)**, which is an aspect of peripheral vision, the ability to see gradual changes in visual texture and larger objects in the visual field. The sine-wave grating is the stimulus used in testing contrast sensitivity **(p. 51)** not the Snellen chart, which is used to test acuity for distant objects **(p. 49–50)**.

3.2   The answer is **D.** Peripheral vision declines by 67% by age 75 **(p. 51)**. The flicker fusion threshold declines with aging **(p. 52)** such that it takes a lower number of flickers of light to be perceived as a continuous light **(p. 51)**. Dynamic visual acuity is the ability to identify a finely detailed target in motion **(p. 52)**. Dynamic visual acuity declines with aging and has been correlated with an increased number of traffic accidents.

3.3   The answer is **D.** All of these changes occur with aging. Peripheral vision declines by 67% by age 75 **(p. 51)**. The ability to distinguish hues

Perceptual Changes With Aging 13

declines with age, especially by age 70, and is greater in the blue-green end of the spectrum than in the red end of the spectrum **(p. 53)**. Loss of sensitivity to higher frequencies occurs with increasing age, with 25% of persons age 65 reporting difficulty with hearing **(p. 54)**.

3.4 The answer is **E**. The intensity of the taste stimulus is thought to be dependent on the number of taste receptors stimulated **(p. 55)**. The large variability between individuals in taste perception not accounted for by age suggests that other factors (health, hormones, genetic variability) may be more important than age in determining taste receptor density and pattern **(p. 55)**.

3.5 The answer is **E**. These changes restrict the amplitude of membrane response and, with the decline in receptors and neurons, result in a less precise initial signal for the auditory system. The atrophy of the stria vascularis decreased the ability of the chochlea to generate a response at all frequencies **(p. 54)**.

CHAPTER 4

Neuroanatomy and Neuropathology of Aging

QUESTIONS

Directions: Select the single best response for each of the following questions:

4.1 The weight of the adult human brain is composed of
   A. Glia (astrocytes, oligodendroglia, and ependyma).
   B. Myelin.
   C. Blood vessels.
   D. All of these.
   E. None of these.

4.2 The synapse permits the directional flow of information
   A. From sensory neuron to motor neuron.
   B. From motor neuron to sensory neuron.
   C. To synaptic vesicles.
   D. To the increased density of the plasma membrane.
   E. None of these.

Directions: For each of the statements below, one or more of the answers is correct. Choose

   A. If 1, 2, and 3 are correct.
   B. If only 1 and 3 are correct.
   C. If only 2 and 4 are correct.
   D. If only 4 is correct.
   E. If all are correct.

4.3 The cardinal lesions of Alzheimer's disease include
1. Neuritic or Alzheimer's plaques.
2. Neurofibrillary tangles.
3. Granulovacuolar degeneration.
4. Overgrowth of astrocytes.

4.4 *Binswanger's disease* is the term applied to
1. Cerebral arteriosclerosis.
2. Multiple microinfarcts.
3. Diffuse pallor of myelin.
4. Unpaired neurofibrillary tangle formation.

ANSWERS

4.1 The answer is **D**. The adult human brain weights 1350 grams and is composed of glia, myelin, and blood vessels **(p. 61)**.

4.2 The answer is **A**. The synapse is a specialized anatomical locus that permits the directional flow of "information" from sensory neurons to motor neurons and never in reverse **(p. 63)**. The polarity of a synapse is identified by the presence of synaptic vesicles. The postsynaptic processes are characterized by an increased density of the plasma membrane **(p. 63)**.

4.3 The answer is **A**. Neuritic plaques, neurofibrillary tangles, and granulovacuolar degeneration are the cardinal features of Alzheimer's disease **(p. 65)**. In Pick's disease (lobar sclerosis) the cortex is severely depleted of neurons and heavily populated with an overgrowth of astrocytes **(p. 68)**.

4.4 The answer is **A**. Approximately 15% of institutionalized individuals with severe dementia will have multiple small cerebral infarcts at postmortem examination **(p. 69)**. The term *Binswanger's disease* has been applied to the morphological constellation of cerebral arteriosclerosis, multiple microinfarcts, and a diffuse pallor of myelin **(p. 69)**.

CHAPTER 5

Chemical Messengers

QUESTIONS

Directions: **Select the single best response for each of the following questions:**

5.1 A chemical neurotransmitter
   A. Is a biomolecule.
   B. Is released across the synapse.
   C. Binds to a receptor that produces a discrete physiologic change
   D. All of these.
   E. None of these.

5.2 The principal inhibitory neurotransmitter in mammalian brains is
   A. Acetylcholine.
   B. The amino acid GABA (γ-aminobutyric acid).
   C. Dopamine.
   D. Serotonin.
   E. None of these.

5.3 The following is true of dopamine (DA) receptors:
   A. They have two classes, D_1 and D_2 receptor subtypes.
   B. The D_1 receptor is predominantly postsynaptic and stimulates adenylate cyclase activity and phosphoinositide turnover.
   C. The D_2 receptor is found at both postsynaptic sites and on axons, dendrites, and soma of presynaptic, DA-producing neurons (autoreceptors) and inhibits adenylate activity and calcium channel passages and potassium conductance.
   D. All of these.
   E. None of these.

5.4 The following is true of glutamic acid (GLU), an excitatory amino acid neurotransmitter:
   A. It has three distinct groups.
   B. It recognizes only aspartate.
   C. The third GLU receptor subtype is similar to muscarinic acetylcholinergic receptors.
   D. Various GLU receptor subtypes are particularly enriched in the hippocampus.
   E. None of these.

Directions: **For each of the statements below, one or more of the answers is correct. Choose**

   A. If 1, 2, and 3 are correct.
   B. If only 1 and 3 are correct.
   C. If only 2 and 4 are correct.
   D. If only 4 is correct.
   E. If all are correct.

5.5 Characteristics of cholinergic neurons include
   1. Nicotinic and muscarinic receptor types.
   2. Septal neurons that project to the hippocampus.
   3. A diagonal band of the nucleus basalis region that projects to the entire cortex.
   4. Decrease in cholinergic neurons in the nucleus basalis in Alzheimer's disease.

5.6 The GABA receptor
   1. Is linked to a second messenger.
   2. Produces inhibition by hyperpolarization of postsynaptic neurons through increase in the permeability of chloride ions.
   3. Decreases calcium or increases potassium ion channel conduction.
   4. Is interacted with by benzodiazepine anxiolytic drugs, barbiturates, and ethanol.

5.7 Catecholamine neurotransmitters include
   1. Dopamine.
   2. Norepinephrine.
   3. Epinephrine.
   4. Serotonin.

Chemical Messengers 19

5.8 The following is true of the indolamine, serotonin (5-hydroxytryptamine [5-HT]):
1. It has three types of receptors: 5-HT_1, 5-HT_2, 5-HT_3.
2. 13 molecular subtypes of 5-HT receptors have been identified to date.
3. These subtypes all appear to be linked to second messengers via G protein.
4. The actual second messengers and the effect of the receptor is consistent for each subtype of 5-HT receptor.

5.9 Neuropeptides are grouped
1. By size.
2. By receptor activity.
3. By prohormone.
4. By similarity of physiological effect.

ANSWERS

5.1 The answer is **D**. A chemical neurotransmitter has these three characteristics **(p. 73)**.

5.2 The answer is **B (p. 78)**. The inhibitory effect of GABA is mediated by two distinct receptor subtypes: GABA-A and GABA-B **(p. 78)**.

5.3 The answer is **D (p. 80)**. Stimulant drugs (cocaine, amphetamine, methylphenidate) inhibit the reuptake of DA in the synaptic cleft by the DA transport system. The classical antipsychotic drugs block D_2 dopamine receptors by binding to the DA recognition site **(p. 80)**.

5.4 The answer is **D**. GLU receptors were classified originally on the basis of whether they would or would not bind the N-methyl-D-aspartate (NMDA) analog. Today these GLU receptors have been divided into five distinct groups **(p. 84)**. The NMDA receptors recognize aspartate as well as GLU and contain at least four other functional subcomponents, making it similar to the benzodiazepine/GABA receptor complex **(p. 84)**. The fifth GLU receptor subtype is linked to the IP3/DAG second messenger single transduction pathway and represents a membrane receptor more like the muscarinic acetylcholine receptor than the nicotine (channel) receptor. The neurons containing the various GLU receptor subtypes are distributed among several regions of the brain and are particularly enriched in the hippocampal subfield **(p. 84)**. The pathological involvement of GLU neurons in stroke, epileptic foci, learning, and memory disorders are a focus of research **(pp. 84–85)**.

5.5 The answer is **D**. The general types of cholinergic receptor have been identified: type I (nicotinic) and type II (muscarinic) **(pp. 77–78)**. Long projections of neurons with acetylcholine as their neurotransmitter are found in the dorsal tegmental nuclei of the midbrain, the magnocellular neurons of the septum, and the diagonal band/nucleus basalis region **(p. 76)**.

5.6 The answer is **C**. The GABA-A receptors produce inhibition by hyperpolarization of the postsynaptic neurons through an increase in the permeability of chloride ion channels **(p. 78)**. GABA-A receptors are similar to nicotinic acetylcholine receptors and produce inhibition by hyperpolarization of the postsynaptic neuron by increasing chloride ion channel permeability. The GABA-B receptor, which resembles the muscarinic acetylcholine receptor, is linked to second messengers and acts by decreasing calcium or increasing potassium ion channel conductance **(p. 78)**. The benzodiazepine anxiolytic drugs, the barbiturates, and ethanol all interact with the GABA-A receptor. This interaction is the physiologic basis for the pharmacological ability of these substances to potentiate each other's effect **(p. 78)**.

5.7 The answer is **A**. Dopamine, norepinephrine, and epinephrine are the three catecholamine neurotransmitters that share a similar molecular structure based on the amino acid tyrosine **(p. 79)**.

5.8 The answer is **A**. The actual second messenger and the effect for the various subtypes of 5-HT receptors (stimulatory or inhibitory) can be quite different **(p. 81)**.

5.9 The answer is **C**. Neuropeptides in the central nervous system are grouped by sequence similarities, receptor activity, and similarity of physiologic effect **(p. 86)**. Examples are the tachykinins, which mediate blood pressure response (substance P, kassinin, eledoisin, bradykinin), and the endogenous opioids (endorphins, enkephalins, and dynorphin), which produce analgesia in neuronal systems associated with pain sensation **(p. 86)**. A larger protein, termed a *prohormone*, is the DNA strand encoding the neuropeptide precursor. It is transcribed into an mRNA sequence within the cell nucleus, and a protein is formed from the prohormone mRNA at the ribosomes and assembled into vesicles at the Golgi apparatus **(p. 86)**.

Chapter 6

Genetics and Geriatric Psychiatry

QUESTIONS

Directions: **Select the single best response for each of the following questions:**

6.1 All of the following are true concerning genetic diseases *except*
   A. The X chromosome contains 112 disease-associated genes.
   B. The Y chromosome contains one disease-associated gene.
   C. The gene for diabetes mellitus is located on chromosome 11.
   D. The gene for Huntington's chorea is found on chromosome 4p16.3.
   E. APOE6 allele is linked with Alzheimer's disease.

6.2 Genetic factors involved in longevity include
   A. The maximum human life span of about 120 years.
   B. Longevity genes that produce free radicals and those that can repair cell damage.
   C. Female advantage due to homogametic sex chromosomes (two X chromosomes).
   D. All of these.
   E. None of these.

6.3 All are true about mitochondrial DNA (mtDNA) *except*
   A. mtDNA are complex, double-stranded circles made up of 16,569 base pairs and are predominately maternally inherited.
   B. mtDNA are vulnerable to damage by oxygen free radicals.
   C. Mutant and normal mtDNA segregate to specific daughter cells.
   D. All of these.
   E. None of these.

Directions: For each of the statements below, one or more of the answers is correct. Choose

- A. If 1, 2, and 3 are correct.
- B. If only 1 and 3 are correct.
- C. If only 2 and 4 are correct.
- D. If only 4 is correct.
- E. If all are correct.

6.4 Syndromes of premature aging include
1. Werner's syndrome (adult progeria)—an autosomal recessive trait of chromosome 8.
2. Hutchinson-Gilford syndrome—an autosomal recessive trait.
3. Down's syndrome—a trisomy of chromosome 21.
4. Aflatoxin syndrome—an autosomal recessive trait of chromosome 3.

6.5 Genetic studies can be divided into
1. Population genetics—twin studies and family studies.
2. Studies of telomeres.
3. Molecular genetics—studying segments of the genome across individuals within a family using restriction fragment length polymorphisms (RFLPs).
4. Medellian genetics.

6.6 Molecular genetic studies have found
1. No evidence for linkage of HLA markers with Alzheimer's disease.
2. An association between apolipoprotein E4 allele (APOE4)—its gene located on chromosome 19—and Alzheimer's disease.
3. Preliminary findings of an association between manic depressive illness and chromosome 11.
4. An association between depression and the X chromosome.

ANSWERS

6.1 The answer is **D (pp. 99, 101–102)**. The APOE4 allele located on chromosome 19 has been liked with Alzheimer's disease **(p. 101)**.

Genetics and Geriatric Psychiatry

6.2 The answer is **D**. When considering genetic factors affecting longevity, these are frequently mentioned **(p. 96)**. Environmental factors (toxins, health habits, and diet) also significantly influence longevity.

6.3 The answer is **C**. When cells divide, both the mutant and the normal mtDNA are randomly scattered into daughter cells **(p. 97)**.

6.4 The answer is **A (pp. 97–98)**. There is no Aflatoxin syndrome. Aflatoxin is a common, potent carcinogen implicated in the development of liver cancer. It is an example of a genetic/environmental interaction that can shorten life expectancy **(p. 98)**.

6.5 The answer is **B (pp. 98–101)**. Using the techniques of twin studies and family studies and the recently developed tools of molecular genetics (e.g., RFLP), specific information about the genetic basis of Huntington's chorea, Alzheimer's disease, and mood disorders are being determined **(pp. 98–101)**.

6.6 The answer is **A (p. 101)**. Although there is a higher prevalence of depression among women age 30–50, there is currently no identified genetic basis for major depressive disorder.

CHAPTER 7

Psychological Aspects of Normal Aging

QUESTIONS

Directions: **Select the single best response for each of the following questions:**

7.1 *Cognition* is the term applied to human intellectual function that includes
   A. Perception, attention, and memory.
   B. Reasoning and decision making.
   C. Problem solving and formation of complex structure of knowledge.
   D. All of these.
   E. None of these.

7.2 The stages involved in the information-processing model include the following *except*
   A. Registration.
   B. Primary memory and secondary memory.
   C. Tertiary memory.
   D. All of these.
   E. None of these.

7.3 The following theoretical models of memory include
   A. The information processing model and episodic/segmental memory model.
   B. The explicit/implicit memory model and the level-of-processing model.
   C. The parallel distribution model.
   D. All of these.
   E. None of these.

7.4 Age-related decline in memory performance is seen in all *except*
   A. Free recall.
   B. Recognition memory.
   C. Secondary memory.
   D. All of these.
   E. None of these.

7.5 Persons age 75 of upper socioeconomic status were found to have about
   A. 1.5 chronic conditions per person.
   B. 2.0 chronic conditions per person.
   C. 2.5 chronic conditions per person.
   D. All of these.
   E. None of these.

7.6 Intellectual performance across the life span includes
   A. Attention, memory, and recall.
   B. Crystalized ability and fluid ability.
   C. Reasoning, decision making, and problem solving.
   D. All of these.
   E. None of these.

7.7 All of the following results have been found in studies of older persons with a battery of neuropsychological tests *except*
   A. Aging affects construction.
   B. Aging affects specific information processing.
   C. Aging affects nonverbal perceptual processing.
   D. Aging affects right hemispheric function.
   E. None of these.

7.8 Studies of persons living to 100 years of age have shown that
   A. There are different paths to longevity.
   B. For some centenarians, strong genetic tendencies or a family history of longevity are important.
   C. For other centenarians, the ability to efficiently adapt to circumstances throughout their lives through problem solving or adaptive personality types are important.
   D. All of these.
   E. None of these.

Psychological Aspects of Normal Aging 27

Directions: **For each of the statements below, one or more of the answers is correct. Choose**

    A. If 1, 2, and 3 are correct.
    B. If only 1 and 3 are correct.
    C. If only 2 and 4 are correct.
    D. If only 4 is correct.
    E. If all are correct.

7.9 Areas included in the psychology of aging include
    1. Experimental and cognitive psychology.
    2. Neuropsychology and personality and social psychology.
    3. Health and behavior.
    4. Longevity and successful aging.

7.10 The capacity of secondary memory to obtain new information with aging is
    1. Affected by aging.
    2. Not affected by aging.
    3. Declines with aging.
    4. Increases with aging.

7.11 The components of attention include
    1. Registration.
    2. Selective attention.
    3. Recall.
    4. Divided attention.

7.12 Factors affecting better mortality and good health with aging include
    1. Systolic blood pressure.
    2. Serum cholesterol.
    3. Upper socioeconomic status.
    4. None of these

7.13 Longitudinal studies of aging include
    1. The Berkeley Growth and Guidance Study follow-up, termed the Berkeley Older Generation Study.
    2. The Seattle Longitudinal Study.
    3. The Baltimore Aging Study.
    4. The Duke Longitudinal Study.

7.14 The decline in peripheral hearing experienced by older people results from
1. The loss of sensitivity to higher auditory frequencies.
2. An increased tendency to recruitment.
3. An increased probability of phonemic regression or decreased speech intelligibility.
4. None of these.

7.15 Factors affecting the older worker include
1. Plant closings.
2. Reductions in the work force.
3. The introduction of new technologies.
4. The reality of up to 40 years of retirement (retiring at age 55 and living to age 95).

7.16 Research into adult personality development has found
1. Greater stability in personality across the adult life cycle.
2. Maintenance of self-esteem at adult levels in later life.
3. That different personality typologies adapt or respond differently to life events.
4. That gender differences are typical.

ANSWERS

7.1 The answer is **D**. All of these factors comprise the range of intellectual functions termed *cognition* **(p. 106)**.

7.2 The answer is **D**. The information-processing model of memory postulates that information flows through a series of stages: registration = sensory memory (preattention and highly unstable); primary memory = short-term memory; secondary memory = long-term memory; and tertiary memory = the repository of well-learned information and personal information **(p. 106)**.

7.3 The answer is **D**. All of these are theoretical models of memory function **(pp. 106–107)**. Clinically, the information-processing model has been used extensively and has the largest amount of data from normal aging and studies of abnormal memory function **(p. 107)**.

7.4 The answer is **B**. Recall tasks of memory decline with age more than recognition tasks **(p. 107)**. Because aging produces a generalized

Psychological Aspects of Normal Aging 29

slowing in all forms of information processing, this slowing also affects memory performance **(p. 107)**.

7.5 The answer is **A**. Persons age 75 of upper socioeconomic status were found to have about 1.5 chronic conditions per person, a number of chronic conditions similar to persons of lower socioeconomic status age 42–43 **(p. 109)**.

7.6 The answer is **B**. Two replicative patterns of intellectual performance across the life span are crystalized abilities and fluid abilities **(p. 108)**. Crystalized ability refers to knowledge acquired in the course of the socialization process that remains stable over the adult life span **(p. 108)**. Fluid ability refers to the abilities involved in the solution of novel problems that tend to decline gradually from youth to old adulthood **(p. 108)**.

7.7 The answer is **D**. Although the neuropsychological and psychometric literature suggest a greater decline in the function of the left hemisphere compared with the right hemisphere, controlled laboratory studies found minimal or no age differences **(p. 111)**. One study of a large sample of normal, older adults found little evidence of decline in cognitive function before age 80 **(p. 111)**. Significant declines in short-term visual memory, serial digit learning, and facial recognition were supported by later studies, which found that these functions (construction, speed of information processing, and nonverbal perceptual processing) were affected by aging **(p. 111)**. This remains an area requiring further study for clarification and explanation of findings.

7.8 The answer is **D**. Studies of centenarians in Hungary, France, Japan, Sweden, Mexico, and the United States found two groups of centenarians with different paths to longevity **(p. 117)**. In one group of centenarians, either high intelligence or problem-solving ability resulted in survival. In another group of centenarians, adaptive personality type was identified as the variable contributing to longevity **(p. 117)**.

7.9 The answer is **E**. These five areas comprise the domains of the psychology of aging: 1) experimental and cognitive psychology, 2) neuropsychology, 3) personality and social psychology, 4) health behavior, and 5) longevity and successful aging **(p. 105)**.

7.10 The answer is **B**. Aging affects secondary memory, producing an age-related decline **(p. 107)**.

7.11 The answer is **C.** In selective attention, the relevant and irrelevant sources of information are defined during the task performance, resulting in attention being selectively focused on the relevant information **(p. 108)**. With divided attention, multiple sources of information are relevant and must be attended to simultaneously **(p. 108)**.

7.12 The answer is **A.** A study of healthy 60-year-olds followed until age 80 found that systolic blood pressure and serum cholesterol levels were associated with good health at age 80 **(p. 109)**. Persons age 75 of upper socioeconomic status had the same number of chronic conditions (1.5) as persons age 42–43 with lower socioeconomic status **(p. 109)**.

7.13 The answer is **E.** Although different populations are sampled, these studies have followed a cohort of community residents longitudinally (the Seattle Longitudinal Study **(pp. 108, 114)**, the Baltimore Longitudinal Study **(p. 109)**, the Duke Longitudinal Study **(p. 108)**. The Berkeley Generation Study is a follow-up study of 420 men and women initially interviewed in 1928–1929 as parents of children involved in the Berkeley Growth and Guidance Study **(p. 114)**.

7.14 The answer is **E.** Presbycusis is a major cause of age-related peripheral hearing decline **(p. 110)**.

7.15 The answer is **E.** These factors require considerable change in the concept of aging and in the funding of retirement **(p. 113)**.

7.16 The answer is **E.** All personality patterns are not associated with the same consequences **(p. 113)**. Patterns characterized by better adjustment in earlier life may lead to more positive outcomes in later life **(p. 113)**.

CHAPTER 8

Social and Economic Factors Related to Psychiatric Disorders in Late Life

QUESTIONS

Directions: **Select the single best response for each of the following questions:**

8.1 Social risk factors involved in Stage V of the Social Precursors of Psychiatric Disorders Model include
  A. Chronic stressor (vulnerability) and social support (protective factors).
  B. Early events and achievements.
  C. Occupation, income, and marital status.
  D. All of these.
  E. None of these.

8.2 Psychiatric disorders may be measured by
  A. Diagnostic instruments (e.g., Research Diagnostic Criteria) and symptom measures.
  B. Self-report of past diagnoses.
  C. Chart review.
  D. All of these.
  E. None of these.

8.3 Depressive symptoms and depressive illness in late life have been found to be associated with
  A. Poverty and chronic illness.
  B. Cognitive impairment.
  C. Disability measurement in terms of Activities of Daily Living (ADL).
  D. All of these.
  E. None of these.

8.4 When the relationship between social support and psychiatric disorders (not depression) was studied, it was found that
   A. Older persons with schizophrenia in the community had smaller social networks than younger persons with schizophrenia.
   B. The major support of persons with schizophrenia with mild symptoms was their family compared with persons with severe symptoms who relied primarily on nonfamily members.
   C. Persons with late-onset alcohol problems had smaller social networks than their peers.
   D. All of these.
   E. None of these.

8.5 The social precursors of psychiatric disorders include
   A. Demographic variables, early events, and achievements.
   B. Later events and achievements and social integration.
   C. Vulnerability or protective factors, provoking agents, and coping.
   D. All of these.
   E. None of these.

Directions: **For each of the statements below, one or more of the answers is correct. Choose**

   A. If 1, 2, and 3 are correct.
   B. If only 1 and 3 are correct.
   C. If only 2 and 4 are correct.
   D. If only 4 is correct.
   E. If all are correct.

8.6 Data from age-heterogeneous studies can be used to determine
   1. The role of age as a risk factor for the development of psychiatric disorders.
   2. How social factors operate during later life.
   3. Whether other risk factors vary in direction or magnitude across age groups.
   4. How gender differences in late life affect the prevalence of psychiatric disorders.

8.7 Data from family caregivers of demented older adults
1. Provide specific data on the impact of chronic stress that can lead to psychiatric problems.
2. Provide the best data on the effects of caregiver burden on psychiatric morbidity.
3. Have found that 30%–50% of caregivers of demented elderly meet DSM-III criteria for depression.
4. Suggest high levels of symptoms of anxiety.

8.8 In the United States, federal programs for the elderly include
1. Social Security retirement benefits.
2. Health care financing (Medicare and Medicaid).
3. Disability benefits.
4. Food stamps.

ANSWERS

8.1 The answer is **A**. Social support versus social isolation and chronic stress were identified in Stage V of the Social Precursors of Psychiatric Disorders Model **(p. 131)**.

8.2 The answer is **A**. Two dimensions have been used to measure psychiatric disorders: diagnostic criteria such as the Research Diagnostic Criteria (first dimension) and symptom measures (second dimension) **(pp. 132–133)**.

8.3 The answer is **D**. The literature documents a clear and strong relationship between these factors and the presence of depressive symptoms and depression **(p. 136)**.

8.4 The answer is **D**. The severity of schizophrenia (mild or severe) affected the type of social support (family versus nonfamily) used **(p. 138)**. Persons with late-onset alcoholism were found to have smaller social networks than their nondrinking age mates **(p. 138)**.

8.5 The answer is **E**. The theoretical model of the Social Precursors of Psychiatric Disorders **(Table 8–1, p. 131)** resulted from research in the areas of social science, epidemiology, and social psychiatry **(p. 130)** and includes the six stages discussed **(pp. 131–132)**.

8.6 The answer is **B.** Heterogeneous age samples (e.g., all adults age 18 and older) provide valuable information about the role of age as a risk factor for psychiatric disorder and whether other risk factors vary in direction or magnitude across age groups **(p. 133)**.

8.7 The answer is **A.** Studies of family caregivers of demented adults provided specific information on the impact of the chronic stressor of caregiving on the development of psychiatric illness **(p. 137)**. Some 30%–50% of these caregivers were found to develop a depressive disorder **(p. 137)**.

8.8 The answer is **E.** Income maintenance and health care financing are the two areas of federal programs for the elderly **(p. 148)**. Income maintenance has been provided in Social Security benefits augmented by disability benefits and food stamps. Medicare for the elderly and Medicaid for the poor are the major health care financing programs of the United States **(p. 148)**.

CHAPTER 9

Epidemiology of Psychiatric Disorders in Late Life

QUESTIONS

Directions: **Select the single best response for each of the following questions:**

9.1 The epidemiology of psychiatric disorders in late life
   A. Is the study of cohorts.
   B. Is the study of risk factors for psychiatric disorders.
   C. Is the comparative study of outcomes.
   D. All of these.
   E. None of these.

9.2 Factors contributing to uncertainty in clinical decision making in the evaluation of the impaired elder adult result from
   A. Problems in the identification of a case.
   B. Differences in observers' ability to detect symptoms and signs of disorder.
   C. Knowledge of the relationship between normality and disease and lack of data about the natural history of the disorder.
   D. All of these.
   E. None of these.

9.3 Psychiatric epidemiologic studies can contribute to the mental health of older adults by
   A. Identifying cases and revealing the distribution of psychiatric disorders in the elderly.
   B. Tracing historical trends in mental illness and determining the etiology of psychiatric disorder in later life.
   C. Examining the use of psychiatric and other mental health services by the elderly.
   D. All of these.
   E. None of these.

9.4 Specific approaches used to identify cases by psychiatric epidemiologic studies include
   A. Chart review, the use of established case registries, and self-administered symptoms scales and personality inventories.
   B. The use of standardized interviews.
   C. Clinician review of data from a survey questionnaire assigning a diagnoses based on recorded data from the interview.
   D. All of these.
   E. None of these.

9.5 Epidemiologic studies have found the following associations *except*
   A. First-degree relatives of Alzheimer's disease patients with aphasia and agraphia have a 44% increased risk of developing senile dementia by age 90.
   B. An association between Alzheimer's disease and Down's syndrome, lymphoma, and immune system diatheses.
   C. An association between an impaired memory score and decreased blood levels of Vitamin C and folic acid in well-functioning elderly.
   D. An association between the deletion of the long arm of chromosome 3 and depressive disorder.
   E. None of these.

9.6 The elderly were found
   A. To be less likely to use community-based psychiatric services compared with any other age group.
   B. To be more likely to use psychotropic medication.
   C. To be more likely to visit their primary care physician for treatment of their psychiatric symptoms or disorder.
   D. All of these.
   E. None of these.

Directions: **For each of the statements below, one or more of the answers is correct. Choose**

   A. **If 1, 2, and 3 are correct.**
   B. **If only 1 and 3 are correct.**
   C. **If only 2 and 4 are correct.**
   D. **If only 4 is correct.**
   E. **If all are correct.**

9.7 Epidemiology requires an understanding of the population at risk. Characteristics of persons age 65 and older in the 1990s include
   1. Life expectancy for men is 71 years and for women is 78 years.
   2. Older men more than older women were involved in more stressful and physically demanding occupations and smoked cigarettes.
   3. A rapid increase in persons age 85 and older, which comprise 15% of persons age 65 and older by 2000.
   4. The aging of the baby boomer cohort resulting in a doubling of the number of persons age 65 and older between 1995 and 2030.

9.8 The definition of a case of psychiatric disorder has varied depending on the perspective of the person defining a case. Definitions of a case of psychiatric disorders include
   1. Severity of symptoms.
   2. Physical, psychological, and social impairment secondary to psychiatric symptoms.
   3. Improvement or maintenance of physical function.
   4. The need for "fuzzy sets" (of criteria for a case definition of a specific disorder) to address the cooccurrence in the elderly of more than one disorder simultaneously (e.g., depression and Alzheimer's disease).

9.9 Epidemiologic studies that consider factors *causing* disease consider whether factors
   1. Predispose persons to developing psychiatric disorder.
   2. Document family history.
   3. Precipitate psychiatric disorders.
   4. Demonstrate a longitudinal course of symptoms.

9.10 Epidemiologic studies of older persons resident in the community found
   1. A prevalence of moderate to severe dementia of 4%–6% among community-resident elders and a 50% prevalence rate of moderate and severe dementia among institutionalized elderly.
   2. A 5% prevalence rate of organic brain syndrome or dementia.
   3. A prevalence rate of <1% for major depressive disorder in the elderly and a 15% prevalence rate of depressive symptoms in the elderly.
   4. A prevalence rate of schizophrenic disorders of approximately 0.1%, and a 1.8% prevalence rate for new onset alcoholism for men and approximately 0.3% for women.

ANSWERS

9.1 The answer is **E**. The epidemiology of psychiatric disorders in late life is the study of the distribution of psychiatric disorders among the elderly and the factors that influence the observed distribution **(p. 155)**.

9.2 The answer is **D**. All of these factors contribute to the uncertainty in clinical decision making **(p. 155)**. The older patient may not express or report symptoms traditionally associated with psychiatric diagnoses, and observers may differ in their identification of anxiety in the elderly **(p. 155)**.

9.3 The answer is **D**. Psychiatric epidemiologic studies contribute to the clarification of mental disorders in the elderly by 1) clarifying the specific symptoms of depression in community-resident elderly and hospitalized elderly, 2) identifying the prevalence and incidence of dementia, 3) describing historical trends in the incidence of suicide over the last 10 years and characterizing those at risk, 4) clarifying whether social factors or genetic factors contribute to late-life psychiatric disorder, and 5) characterizing the utilization of psychiatric services by the psychiatrically impaired elderly **(pp. 156–157)**.

9.4 The answer is **D**. Following the establishment of the criteria for case identification, one of these approaches is used **(p. 158)**. Standardized scales (e.g., the Center for Epidemiologic Studies of Depression Scale [CES-D]) are effective screening instruments for community populations but lack the diagnostic specificity of standardized instruments based on a diagnostic system **(p. 158)**.

9.5 The answer is **D**. There are no studies that have shown an association between chromosome 3 and depressive disorder. The association between Alzheimer's disease and Down's syndrome, the increased risk for the development of dementia of the Alzheimer's type (DAT) by first-degree relatives of persons with DAT, and the role of nutrients in memory function have been well studied **(pp. 164–165)**.

9.6 The answer is **D**. Older adults with psychiatric symptoms and disorders were shown in several studies to underutilize psychiatric services and to visit their primary care provider for mental health care **(pp. 166–168)**.

9.7 The answer is **E**. The aging of the baby boomer cohort and the rapid increase among persons age 85 and older are changing the composition of the older population of the United States and increasing the size of

Epidemiology of Psychiatric Disorders in Late Life

the population at risk for the development of the psychiatric disorders of late adult life **(p. 156)**.

9.8 The answer is **E**. Although some emphasize diagnostic criteria that specify the symptoms of the psychiatric, psychological, and social impairment resulting from the psychiatric disorder, clinicians may be more inclined to "treat the disease" than "to improve function" **(p. 157)**. In contrast, family members often are more concerned about improved function than about symptom remission **(p. 157)**.

9.9 The answer is **B**. Factors that either predispose individuals to developing psychiatric disorders or precipitate such disorders are termed *etiologic factors* **(p. 164)**. Population-based studies provide information on both genetic and environmental causative agents **(p. 164)**. Studies of risk factors for Alzheimer's disease are an example of how the epidemiologic studies have identified etiologic agents **(p. 165)**.

9.10 The answer is **E**. The prevalence of psychiatric disorders in community-resident elderly have been found to vary based on the specific disorder **(pp. 159–162)**. The distinction between the prevalence of depressive symptoms, particularly among the medically ill, versus the prevalence of depressive disorder in the elderly is an important one **(pp. 161–162, Tables 9–4 and 9–5)**.

Section II

The Diagnostic Interview in Late Life

CHAPTER 10

The Psychiatric Interview of the Geriatric Patient

QUESTIONS

Directions: **Select the single best response for each of the following questions:**

10.1 In order to obtain the historical information
   A. The caregiver should be interviewed first.
   B. Family members should be interviewed first.
   C. The older patient should be interviewed first.
   D. All of these.
   E. None of these.

10.2 A structured review of the more important psychiatric symptoms is a crucial component of the psychiatric interview of the geriatric patient because
   A. It screens for psychiatric disorders.
   B. The older adult may attribute symptoms and signs of treatable psychiatric disorders to "getting older."
   C. It is an effective way of conveying the physician's role as healer.
   D. All of these.
   E. None of these.

10.3 Specific parts of the psychiatric interview of the geriatric patient include all *except*
   A. A description of current symptoms and a review of past medical and psychiatric disorders.
   B. Family history and review of all medications taken currently and in the past and their effects.
   C. Treatment contract.
   D. All of these.
   E. None of these.

10.4 Screens to assess the presence of cognitive impairment and dementia include
   A. Short Portable Mental Status Questionnaire (SPMSQ).
   B. Mini-Mental State Exam (MMSE).
   C. Blessed Dementia Index.
   D. All of these.
   E. None of these.

Directions: **For each of the statements below, one or more of the answers is correct. Choose**

   A. If 1, 2, and 3 are correct.
   B. If only 1 and 3 are correct.
   C. If only 2 and 4 are correct.
   D. If only 4 is correct.
   E. If all are correct.

10.5 Factors influencing an older person's definition of illness include
   1. The historical background and values of the older person.
   2. The older person's social class.
   3. The cultural background of the older person.
   4. The level of discomfort produced by the illness.

10.6 Self-administered scales to assess the presence of depressive symptoms used in community resident elderly include
   1. The Zung Self-Rated Depression Scale.
   2. The Geriatric Depression Scale (GDS).
   3. The Carroll Rating Scale for Depression.
   4. The Center for Epidemiologic Studies Depression Scale (CES-D).

10.7 The factors identified in a factor analysis of the CES-D in a community population were
   1. An enervation factor.
   2. A positive affect factor.
   3. An interpersonal relationship factor.
   4. A combined melancholic factor.

The Psychiatric Interview of the Geriatric Patient

10.8 Rating scales and standardized or structured interviews are both incorporated into the diagnostic assessment of psychiatric patients
1. To provide a standard means of describing change in clinical status.
2. To provide information on specific factors associated with given psychiatric disorders.
3. To provide systematic, reproducible diagnoses for third-party carriers.
4. To provide information on outcomes.

10.9 Structured clinical interviews include
1. Present State Examination (PSE).
2. Structured Clinical Interview for the DSM-IV (SCID).
3. Diagnostic Interview Schedule (DIS).
4. Sandoz Clinical Assessment-Geriatric (SCAG).

10.10 Approaches facilitating communication with the older patient include
1. Addressing the older person by his or her given name and sitting within arm's length of the person.
2. Speaking clearly and slowly in simple sentences and pacing the interview to give the older person time to respond.
3. Using nonverbal communication to convey concern and attention to the older person's comments and statements.
4. Communicating a willingness to continue working with the older patient.

ANSWERS

10.1 The answer is **C**. An attempt should be made to interview the older patient first. If possible, permission can be obtained from the patient to interview family members. This approach indicates respect for the older person regardless of the cognitive or physical capacities of the older person **(p. 175)**.

10.2 The answer is **B**. The older patient may exhibit an attitudinal bias toward aging. "I guess I'm just getting old and there's nothing really to worry about. Most people slow down when they get older." Such attitudes may result in an underreporting of psychiatric symptoms and disorders **(p. 176)**.

10.3   The answer is **C**. A treatment contract is completed following an evaluation and discussion of the results with the patient. The specific parts of the psychiatric interview of the older patient are summarized on Table 10–1 **(p. 176)**.

10.4   The answer is **D**. The SPMSQ, a 10-question scale, has been used clinically to screen community-resident elderly for the presence of cognitive impairment **(p. 182)**. The 30-item MMSE assesses the additional domains of calculation, recall, and language **(p. 182)**. Because of the frequent presence of multiple small infarcts with primary degenerative dementia, the Hachinski Scale has had limited clinical usefulness **(p. 183)**. The Blessed Dementia Index is one clinical assessment tool for the staging of dementia. The total score of the Blessed Dementia Index, which requires the use of clinical judgement, was found to correlate with cerebral changes **(p. 183)**.

10.5   The answer is **E**. As the United States population becomes more diverse, the cultural background and values in the context of social class are and will be important factors that affect the older person's definition of illness **(p. 176)**. The level of discomfort experienced by the older person will determine whether the older person decides to seek treatment **(p. 176)**.

10.6   The answer is **D**. The CES-D is the most widely used screening instrument for depression in community-resident elderly because of the normative population data **(p. 183)**. The GDS developed specifically to screen older persons for the presence of depressive symptoms with a forced choice format (Yes or No) has not been used in community populations and is not well standardized **(pp. 183–184)**. The Carroll Rating Scale for Depression based on the Hamilton Depression Scale has not been used extensively in the elderly **(p. 184)**.

10.7   The answer is **A**. An enervation factor, a positive affect factor, and an interpersonal relationship factor were the three factors identified by a factor analysis of the CES-D based on community population **(p. 183)**. A combined melancholic factor was not found **(p. 183)**.

10.8   The answer is **B**. The use of rating scales and standardized or structured interviews has provided important information on diagnoses and change in clinical status that has proved useful for third-party carriers **(p. 182)**.

10.9   The answer is **A**. The Sandoz Clinical Assessment—Geriatric (SCAG) is an 18-item symptom scale that rates each symptom on a 7-point scale.

Its usefulness in discriminating between subgroups of psychiatrically disturbed older adults remains to be tested. The SCAG is an assessment scale **(p. 184)**. The PSE is not an interview but a list of definitive behaviors or symptoms of psychiatric disorders that are rated by a clinician as present or absent. A computer algorithm provides a diagnosis **(p. 185)**. The PSE focuses on 1 month before the evaluation and uses the *International Classification of Disease* (ICD), not the DSM, to make diagnoses. The SCID is the most frequently used instrument in the United States and is easily adapted to the Research Diagnostic Criteria (RDC) and DSM-IV. Interviewers using the SCID have the flexibility to add additional questions and to use all available data to assign diagnoses **(p. 186)**. The DIS, which can be administered by a lay interviewer, is a highly structured, computer-scored interview that allows psychiatric diagnoses to be made according to DSM-IV criteria, Feighner criteria, or RDC. The DIS has been used in clinical studies and community-based studies including the Epidemiologic Catchment Area study **(p. 186)**.

10.10 The answer is **E**. Use of the older person's surname conveys respect. Adjusting speech for the older person with hearing impairment will facilitate communication. Pacing the interview to include silences gives the older person the opportunity to formulate answers to questions and to elaborate on points he or she wishes to make to convey an understanding of the reality of the functional status of the elderly **(p. 187)**. The clinician can use nonverbal communication to demonstrate his or her concern and empathy with the older person. Persons age 65 and older value loyalty and continuity. The clinician's willingness to continue to work as a professional with the older person has important meaning to the older patient **(p. 187)**.

Chapter 11

Use of the Laboratory in the Diagnostic Workup of Older Adults

QUESTIONS

Directions: **Select the single best response for each of the following questions:**

11.1 The specificity of a test is best described as
   A. The number of persons who have a disorder and who have a positive test result divided by the total number of individuals who have the disorder.
   B. The number of persons who do *not* have a disorder and have a negative test result divided by the total number of persons who do *not* have the disorder.
   C. The proportion of patients with positive test results who have the disorder.
   D. All of these.
   E. None of these.

11.2 The components of the polysomnogram include
   A. Sleep electroencephalogram (EEG).
   B. Electrooculogram.
   C. The submental electromyogram.
   D. All of these.
   E. None of these.

11.3 The electrocardiogram (ECG) is helpful in monitoring the effect of
   A. Antianxiety medications.
   B. Neuroleptic medications.
   C. Tricyclic antidepressants.
   D. All of these.
   E. None of these.

11.4 The thyrotropin-releasing hormone (TRH) stimulation tests
   A. Is an important component of the routine clinical workup of the depressed or demented older adult.
   B. Is useful in the diagnosis of mania.
   C. Requires a 24-hour fast and a 14-day drug-free period.
   D. All of these.
   E. None of these.

11.5 All of the following are true *except*
   A. Computed tomography (CT) provides a structural assessment of cerebral atrophy, ventricular size, and estimation of the amount of cerebrospinal fluid.
   B. Using positron-emitting radioisotopes, magnetic resonance imaging (MRI) provides functional information about cerebral perfusion and metabolism associated with perception, learning, and recall.
   C. Positron-emission tomography (PET) using ^{18}F-labeled 2-deoxy-2-fluoro-D-glucose found decreased metabolic action in temporal and parietal regions of patients with Alzheimer's disease and decreased glucose utilization in epileptogenic foci in 70% of patients with partial seizure disorders.
   D. Single-photon emission computerized tomography (SPECT) provides information on brain and organ function and is less costly than PET.
   E. None of these.

11.6 EEG sleep studies found that patients with psychotic depression
   A. Had marked initial insomnia.
   B. Had an increased percentage of Stage 1 sleep.
   C. Had long rapid eye movement (REM) latencies.
   D. All of these.
   E. None of these.

11.7 Neuropsychological evaluation can
   A. Assist in the diagnosis of brain injury or disease, including localization of the injury, and aid in the determination of the cause of the brain dysfunction.
   B. Track changes in function over time.
   C. Assist in the planning and evaluation in rehabilitation.
   D. All of these.
   E. None of these.

Use of the Laboratory in the Diagnostic Workup of Older Adults 51

Directions: For each of the statements below, one or more of the answers is correct. Choose

- A. If 1, 2, and 3 are correct.
- B. If only 1 and 3 are correct.
- C. If only 2 and 4 are correct.
- D. If only 4 is correct.
- E. If all are correct.

11.8 Laboratory tests are useful
1. To screen and to confirm diagnoses.
2. To confirm the presence of a disease.
3. To predict the patient's response to therapy.
4. To identify those persons most at risk of developing a specific disease.

11.9 Shelps and Schechter suggested nine methodological criteria to use to determine if a diagnostic test is useful as a marker of an illness. These criteria include
1. The presence of a gold standard.
2. Definition of sensitivity and specificity of the test.
3. A clear statement of the limitations of test use.
4. Specification of techniques for ensuring patient comfort.

11.10 Indications for the use of a laboratory test include
1. Unusual symptoms and signs found on examination.
2. An older patient.
3. Illness beginning after ages 40–45.
4. The presence of depressive symptoms.

11.11 Reversible dementias are due to
1. B_{12} deficiency.
2. Substance abuse.
3. Infection.
4. Thyroid dysfunction.

11.12 Components of the thyroid panel include
1. Direct assay of thyroxine (T_4) by radioimmunoassay.
2. Triiodothyronine (T_3) uptake.
3. Calculation of free thyroxin index.
4. The level of thyroid-stimulating hormone (TSH).

11.13 False-positive results of the Dexamethasone Suppression Test (DST) can be caused by
1. Medication (phenytoin, barbiturates, carbamazepine).
2. Endocrine factors (Cushing's disease or pregnancy).
3. Metabolic problems (recent withdrawal from alcohol, rapid weight loss, malnutrition, or nausea and vomiting).
4. Multiinfarct dementia and increased intracranial pressure.

11.14 The advantages of MRI include
1. No radiation is involved.
2. No contrast dye is needed.
3. Its production of high-resolution images distinguishes normal from abnormal.
4. It can obtain pictures from parts of the body usually not accessible by CT scan.

11.15 The comprehensive evaluation of cognitive function can be completed by
1. The Halstead-Reitan Neuropsychological Test Battery.
2. The Weschler Adult Intelligence Scale—Revised (WAIS-R).
3. The Luria-Nebraska Neuropsychological Battery.
4. The Weschler Memory Scale—Revised (WMS-R).

11.16 Personality Assessment Instruments include
1. Minnesota Multiphasic Personality Inventory (MMPI).
2. MMPI-2.
3. Millon Clinical Multiaxial Inventory I (MCMI-I).
4. MCMI-II.

11.17 Projective tests
1. Use a relatively unstructured task that requires individuals to provide the structure.
2. Have weak psychometric properties.
3. May be clinically useful when administered by an experienced and skilled examiner.
4. Include the Rorschach and Thematic Apperception Test.

Use of the Laboratory in the Diagnostic Workup of Older Adults 53

ANSWERS

11.1 The answer is **B**. The specificity of a test is defined as the number of persons who do *not* have the disease and who have a negative test result divided by the total number of individuals who do not have the disorder **(p. 192)**.

11.2 The answer is **D**. The electrooculogram measures eye movements during sleep and the submental electromyogram measures ventilatory air exchange and respiratory effort. These and the sleep EEG comprise the three basic recording variables of the polysomnogram **(p. 194)**.

11.3 The answer is **C**. In near or therapeutic plasma levels, tricyclic antidepressants are associated with a prolonged PR interval and prolonged QRS complex **(p. 194)**. Frequent ECG monitoring of older patients with preexisting bundle branch block is indicated because of the danger of AV or HV block **(p. 194)**.

11.4 The answer is **A**. The TRH test is the most sensitive of the clinical tests for thyroid disorder **(p. 195)**. Patients must fast overnight and be drug free for the previous 7 days **(p. 196)**. The day of the test, the recumbent patient is given 0.5 mg of TRH. The TSH is recorded at 30-minute interviews for 3 hours. A blunted response of TSH to TRH is seen in depressed patients, in functionally euthyroid patients with toxic goiters, and occasionally in patients with pituitary hypothyroidism **(p. 196)**.

11.5 The answer is **B**. MRI is based on the principle that the nuclei of certain atoms (isotopes) behave like spinning magnets. When placed in the static magnetic field of the MRI apparatus, they line up in the direction of that field and wobble randomly. The T_1 time constant is the time required for the nuclei to reach equilibrium in the direction of the field and to wobble randomly **(p. 198)**. The application of a second, right-angle, oscillating field makes the nuclei in the continuous field wobble in unison. T_2 is the time constant for the establishment of the uniform wobbling in the second, right-angle, oscillating magnetic field **(p. 198)**.

11.6 The answer is **E**. Patients with *recent onset depression* were found to have marked initial insomnia, an increased percentage of Stage 1 sleep, and long REM latencies. The sleep of persons with psychotic depression was found to have increased wakefulness, decreased percentage of REM sleep, and decreased REM activity with EEG abnormalities tending to increase with the duration of the illness **(p. 200)**.

11.7 The answer is **D**. Neuropsychologic evaluation is completed by a psychodiagnostics laboratory **(p. 201)**. In addition to testing for the presence and level of severity of specific disorders (neuropsychologic evaluation), services include neuropsychological testing, intelligence testing, and personality testing **(p. 201)**. The proper formulation of the question to be answered by the diagnostician is crucial as it determines which assessment instrument(s) will be used and how best to report the information obtained **(p. 201)**.

11.8 The answer is **B**. Laboratory tests can screen and confirm diagnoses as well as predict the patient's response to therapy **(p. 193)**. Multiple laboratory tests can be helpful if the accumulation of abnormal results confirm the presence of a disorder **(p. 193)**. If only one test is positive and the results of the rest are normal, the use of multiple laboratory tests is less helpful **(p. 193)**.

11.9 The answer is **A**. Although patient comfort is an important concern and can influence the completion of some tests, it was not a specific methodological criteria **(p. 192)**. Additional criteria included a clear definition of "positive" and "negative" results, an independent test (blind to other clinical information), a display of data in useful tabular form; specification of sensitivity and specificity clearly defined and used correctly; limitations of the use of the test clearly stated; and guidelines for the appropriate use of the test, discussion of the cost/benefit ratio of the test, and a description of the procedure for performing the test **(p. 192)**.

11.10 The answer is **A**. Laboratory tests have been helpful and are more likely to be appropriately used in these circumstances **(p. 193)**.

11.11 The answer is **E**. Dementia that are caused by medical conditions that can be treated are termed *reversible dementias*. Thyroid dysfunction, B_{12} deficiency, substance abuse, and infections are examples of reversible dementias **(p. 195)**.

11.12 The answer is **E**. These four tests are helpful in assessing the role of thyroid dysfunction as a cause of depressive symptoms. Subclinical hypothyroidism is a common cause of depressive symptoms in older adults and may be responsive to supplemental thyroid replacement **(p. 195)**.

11.13 The answer is **E**. Medications, endocrine factors, metabolic problems, and neurologic problems can produce false-positive results with the DST test **(p. 196)**.

11.14 The answer is **E**. The disadvantages of the MRI are that it requires the patient to remain perfectly motionless for extended periods in a doughnut-like structure that can produce claustrophic responses in some patients, and the MRI must be housed in a large area devoid of iron and lined in copper **(p. 198)**.

11.15 The answer is **B**. The Halstead-Reitan Neuropsychologic Test Battery is the most widely used and extensively validated battery. Although less established and not as thoroughly researched, the Luria-Nebraska Neuropsychological Battery takes less time to administer, and its content, materials, administration, and scoring are more highly standardized **(p. 203)**. The WAIS-R is a measure of "general" intelligence based on 11 different subtests divided into verbal and performance categories. The WMS-R consists of the Logical Memory and Visual Reproduction subtests of the original instrument and an additional recall trial after a half-hour delay **(p. 203)**.

11.16 The answer is **E**. The MMPI was modified and the MMPI-2 became available in 1989. The MMPI remains the most widely used personality assessment instrument requiring a true-false response to its items **(p. 204)**. The MCMI and its 1987 revision, MCMI-II, another personality inventory, written at an eighth grade level, requires a true-false response to 175 items. The MCMI-II may be used as an efficient "first pass" at personality psychopathological diagnoses of Axis II **(p. 204)**.

11.17 The answer is **E**. These psychodiagnostic tests use vague test stimuli and general instructions that require the individual to provide the structure. Although they possess poor psychometric properties, they continue in widespread use **(p. 205)**. Several scoring systems have been developed for the Rorschach set of 10 cards, but considerable variability in the scoring process remains. The Thematic Apperception Test (TAT) elicits or distinguishes statements about beliefs, attitudes, and motives with the person required to tell a story based on a picture presented by the examiner. Although a formal scoring system is available, the most common method of interpretation is the impressionistic approach **(pp. 205–206)**.

SECTION III

Psychiatric Disorders in Late Life

Chapter 12

Cognitive Disorders

QUESTIONS

Directions: **Select the single best response for each of the following questions.**

12.1 The best term to describe cognitive disorders is
   A. Functional brain disorders.
   B. Organic brain disorders.
   C. Organic brain syndrome.
   D. Senility.
   E. None of these.

12.2 *Dementia* is best defined as
   A. A disorder.
   B. A syndrome.
   C. A category of illness.
   D. All of these.
   E. None of these.

12.3 The course of dementia of the Alzheimer's type (DAT) is
   A. Death within 2 years.
   B. Variable with a range of 5–15 years.
   C. Death within 6 months.
   D. All of these.
   E. None of these.

12.4 All of the following are helpful in identifying depressive pseudodementia *except*
   A. Has a family history of depression.
   B. Exhibits poor motivation.
   C. Frequently gives the answer, "I don't know."
   D. Exhibits aphasia, apraxia, and anomie.
   E. None of these.

12.5 Potentially reversible causes of cognitive impairment are found
   A. Frequently.
   B. Rarely.
   C. In most cases.
   D. All of these.
   E. None of these.

12.6 Evidence of the cholinergic-deficiency hypothesis as the cause of DAT include
   A. The finding in patients with DAT of extensive loss of neurons in the cholinergic nucleus basalis of Meynert.
   B. The identification of the basal forebrain—a major source of choline.
   C. The confirmation of a presynaptic cholinergic deficit in patients with DAT by several studies.
   D. All of these.
   E. None of these.

12.7 DSM-IV criteria for delirium include
   A. Disturbance of consciousness.
   B. Impairment of attention.
   C. Fluctuation of attention.
   D. All of these.
   E. None of these.

12.8 Specific abnormalities in the brains of patients with DAT include
   A. Decreased ability of muscarinic receptors to form a high-affinity agonist state.
   B. Decreased concentration of serotonin and its metabolites.
   C. Neuronal loss in the locus coeruleus (a major source of adrenergic neurons).
   D. All of these.
   E. None of these.

Cognitive Disorders

Directions: For each of the statements below, one or more of the answers is correct. Choose

    A. If 1, 2, and 3 are correct.
    B. If only 1 and 3 are correct.
    C. If only 2 and 4 are correct.
    D. If only 4 is correct.
    E. If all are correct.

12.9 The major features of dementia include
1. Acquired memory impairment.
2. Aphasia, apraxia, and agnosia.
3. Disturbance in executive function.
4. Depression.

12.10 The course of dementia due to head trauma
1. Can show meaningful improvement in cognitive function.
2. Is an inexorable progression to incontinence and loss of cognitive function.
3. Is a stepwise course.
4. Is either stable or can improve over time.

12.11 Other disorders to be ruled out in the presence of dementia include
1. Depression.
2. Delirium.
3. Side effects of medication.
4. Rheumatoid cerebrovasculitis.

12.12 The course of disorders causing dementia vary. Which of the following is correct?
1. Vascular dementia = meaningful improvement over time.
2. Anoxic brain injury = stepwise progression over time.
3. Alzheimer's disease = stable and improved over time.
4. Dementia due to alcohol = slow and insidious progression over time.

12.13 Evidence for the involvement of brain proteins in the pathophysiology of DAT include
1. The presence of soluble beta-amyloid precursor protein (sβPP) in cerebral spinal fluid.
2. Microtubular-associated phosphoprotein tau found in neurofibrillary tangles in a hyperphosporolated form.
3. Identification of the beta-amyloid protein in the posterior brain of persons with DAT.
4. Segregation of point mutations on the amyloid precursor protein (APP) gene on chromosome 21 segregating with DAT in families with familial DAT.

12.14 Specific treatments for DAT include
1. Intravenous muscarinic cholinergic agonist.
2. Tetrahydroaminoacridin (THA), also known as tacrine.
3. Oral administration of choline or lecithin.
4. Intravenous physostigmine.

ANSWERS

12.1 The answer is **E**. As a result of accumulating knowledge, it has become increasingly clear that there is a biologic basis to all behavioral disorders, whether a genetic diathesis or a physiologic change in brain function **(p. 213)**. Thus, all of these terms are obsolete now. Therefore, the broad term *cognitive function* is used in DSM-IV **(p. 213)**.

12.2 The answer is **B**. *Dementia* is best defined as a syndrome, a group of signs and symptoms that cluster together, but that can be caused by a number of underlying diseases **(p. 214)**.

12.3 The answer is **B**. The typical course of DAT from the time of insidious onset ranges from 5–15 years **(p. 214)**.

12.4 The answer is **D**. The term *pseudodementia* has been useful in characterizing impairment that can be caused by depression. Depressive signs and symptoms precede cognitive impairment in this syndrome **(p. 214)**. The presence of aphasia, apraxia, and anomia are seen in the later stages of dementia **(p. 214)**.

12.5 The answer is **B**. Completely reversible cognitive impairment due to correctable causes is rare **(p. 216)**. In one group of unselected elderly

Cognitive Disorders

outpatients, 14% (15 of 107) were identified as having potentially reversible causes of dementia **(p. 216)**, but only 3% (3 of 107) actually returned to normal cognitive function **(p. 217)**.

12.6 The answer is **D**. The cholinergic deficiency has been accepted as the explanation for cognitive decline because of the consistent finding of extensive loss of neurons in the nucleus basalis of Meynert among patients with DAT **(p. 219)**.

12.7 The answer is **D**. The DSM-IV criteria for a diagnosis of delirium also include two other items: a change in cognition or the development of perceptual disturbance; the disturbance of consciousness develops over a short period of time (hours to days), and there is evidence in the database (history, physical examination, or laboratory data) that the disturbance is caused by a general medical condition **(p. 227)**. In the elderly, delirium may occur over a longer period of time due to drugs (e.g., long-acting benzodiazepines) or illness (e.g., renal failure) **(p. 227)**.

12.8 The answer is **D**. These changes are found in the brains of patients with DAT **(pp. 219–220)** and result in the progressive deterioration in memory and eventual change in personality.

12.9 The answer is **A**. The acquired memory impairment termed the *syndrome of dementia* is characterized by an initial, acquired decline in memory. In addition, at least one of the following is required for the diagnosis: aphasia, apraxia, agnosia, disturbance in executive function (planning, organizing, sequencing, and abstracting) **(p. 214)**.

12.10 The answer is **D**. Following an abrupt onset, the course of dementia due to head trauma is either stable or can improve over time **(p. 214)**. The course of DAT is an inexorable progressive deterioration to loss of personality and incontinence. The progression of vascular dementia may be stepwise. If persons with dementia due to alcohol remain free of alcohol, a substantial number will show meaningful improvement in cognitive function **(p. 214)**.

12.11 The answer is **E**. The differential diagnosis of dementia should include depression; delirium **(pp. 214–215)**; and reversible causes of dementia including medication effect, hypothyroidism, subdural hematoma, and rheumatoid cerebrovasculitis **(p. 217)**.

12.12 The answer is **D**. As discussed **(p. 214)**, the course of these dementias vary over time. The course of Alzheimer's disease is slow and insidious in contrast to the course of anoxic brain injury, which is stable. A stepwise course is seen in vascular dementia. In dementia due to alcohol, persons who stop drinking can show meaningful improvement over time **(p. 214)**, arresting the insidious progression.

12.13 The answer is **D**. In a few families with familial DAT, the association of a point mutation on chromosome 21 with the presence of DAT provides evidence for a role of brain proteins, beta-amyloid protein, or another product of amyloid precursor protein (APP) in DAT **(pp. 218–219)**.

12.14 The answer is **B**. The oral administration of precursors of acetylcholine (i.e., lecithin and choline) was ineffective in improving cognitive function **(p. 220)**. Intravenous physostigmine was "modestly helpful" in producing modest improvement in cognitive function in persons with mild dementia **(p. 220)** but was limited in its usefulness because of its short half-life as was the administration of muscarinic cholinergic agonists. Currently, THA is one clinically available treatment for cognitive defects. The oral administration of THA has produced cognitive improvement in a subset of patients with DAT **(p. 221)**.

Chapter 13

Mood Disorders

QUESTIONS

Directions: **Select the single best response for each of the following questions.**

13.1 One study of 1,300 older adults age 60 and older found that

A. 27% had a current major depressive episode.
B. 2% had a current major depressive episode.
C. 0.8% had a current major depressive episode.
D. All of these.
E. None of these.

13.2 The rates of major depressive disorder among elderly nursing home residents range from

A. 12% to 16%.
B. 25% to 30%.
C. 32% to 36%.
D. All of these.
E. None of these.

13.3 Although manic episodes in late life were found to be uncommon by the Epidemiologic Catchment Area survey, the prevalence of bipolar disorders among nursing home residents was found to be

A. 20%.
B. 10%.
C. 5%.
D. All of these.
E. None of these.

13.4 The duration of a major depressive disorder throughout the life cycle is approximately
   A. 18 months.
   B. 9 months.
   C. 3 months.
   D. All of these.
   E. None of these.

13.5 Older adults with major depressive disorder treated with combined interpersonal psychotherapy and nortriptyline had a response rate of
   A. 80%.
   B. 60%.
   C. 40%.
   D. All of these.
   E. None of these.

13.6 When elderly persons with treatment-resistant depression were followed-up 15 months after treatment with an antidepressant and/or electroconvulsive therapy, it was found that
   A. 27% were clinically improved.
   B. 37% were clinically improved.
   C. 47% were clinically improved.
   D. All of these.
   E. None of these.

13.7 Which of the following is a true statement about the dexamethasone suppression test (DST)?
   A. It has proved less reliable in predicting the long-term follow-up of depressed persons.
   B. Nonsuppression of cortisol on DST after the treatment of depression is associated with a higher risk for early relapse.
   C. Baseline DST does not predict response to antidepressant therapy.
   D. All of these.
   E. None of these.

Mood Disorders **67**

13.8 Depressed patients who reported an adequate social support network at the time of the index depressive episodes were

A. 2.3 times more likely to have recovered from depression.
B. 5 times more likely to have recovered from depression.
C. 7.5 times more likely to have recovered from depression.
D. All of these.
E. None of these.

13.9 Precipitants to late-onset mania include

A. Stroke.
B. Head trauma.
C. Other brain insults.
D. All of these.
E. None of these.

13.10 Studies of patients with unipolar depression in late life suggest that the genetic contribution is

A. Stronger.
B. Weaker.
C. Intermediate.
D. All of these.
E. None of these.

13.11 Numerous neurotransmitter and neuroendocrine changes are common to old age and depressive illness. The prevalence of depression in late life was found to be

A. Relatively low.
B. Relatively high.
C. Not different from younger age cohorts.
D. All of these.
E. None of these.

13.12 Elderly patients with bipolar disorder exhibit

A. Elevated mood.
B. Irritable mood.
C. Depressive admixture.
D. All of these.
E. None of these.

13.13 Older African-American men may
 A. Report feelings of sadness.
 B. Report melancholia.
 C. Report feelings of low self-worth.
 D. All of these.
 E. None of these.

13.14 Symptoms of depression not otherwise specified require the presence of symptoms for
 A. More than 2 years.
 B. 2 weeks.
 C. Less than 2 weeks.
 D. All of these.
 E. None of these.

13.15 Somatic symptoms of distress associated with bereavement include
 A. Tightness in the throat.
 B. Shortness of breath.
 C. Sighing respirations.
 D. All of these.
 E. None of these.

13.16 Toxic causes of mood disorder include
 A. Beta-blockers and clonidine.
 B. Benzodiazepines.
 C. Reserpine and methyldopa.
 D. All of these.
 E. None of these.

13.17 The presence of hypochondriacal symptoms and depressive symptoms may be associated with attempted suicide. Among patients with hypochondriacal symptoms, the percentage attempting suicide was found to be
 A. 25%.
 B. 35%.
 C. 45%.
 D. All of these.
 E. None of these.

Mood Disorders **69**

13.18 The diagnosis of depression in a patient with alcohol dependence should not be made until the patient has been sober for at least

    A. 6 weeks.
    B. 4 weeks.
    C. 2 weeks.
    D. All of these.
    E. None of these.

13.19 The psychotherapeutic treatment of depression includes

    A. Family therapy.
    B. Insight-oriented, long-term psychotherapy.
    C. Cognitive behavioral therapy.
    D. All of these.
    E. None of these.

13.20 A therapeutic dose of nortriptyline for an elderly person is

    A. 25–50 mg.
    B. 75–100 mg.
    C. 125–150 mg.
    D. All of these.
    E. None of these.

13.21 The interval between stopping a selective serotonin reuptake inhibitor (SSRI) and starting a monoamine oxidase inhibitor (MAOI) should be

    A. 4–6 weeks.
    B. 2–4 weeks.
    C. 1–2 weeks.
    D. All of these.
    E. None of these.

13.22 Before initiating electroconvulsive therapy (ECT), an MAOI should be stopped

    A. 7 days before treatment.
    B. 10 days before treatment.
    C. 21 days before treatment.
    D. All of these.
    E. None of these.

13.23 To achieve optimal results, the seizure induced with ECT should last
   A. 10 seconds.
   B. 15 seconds.
   C. 25 seconds.
   D. All of these.
   E. None of these.

13.24 When ECT is used in depressed patients who did not respond to antidepressant medication, the response rate is usually
   A. 80% or greater.
   B. 60% or greater.
   C. 40% or greater.
   D. All of these.
   E. None of these.

13.25 When the efficacy of ECT in elderly depressed patients with dementia was studied, it was found that
   A. 86% of patients responded to ECT.
   B. Only 21% experienced a significant worsening of cognition.
   C. 49% of patients treated with ECT showed improved memory function after treatment.
   D. All of these.
   E. None of these.

13.26 Family members play an important role in the evaluation and management of the older depressed patient by
   A. Observing changes in behavior.
   B. Removing possible implements of suicide from easy access.
   C. Facilitating hospitalization for severe symptoms.
   D. All of these.
   E. None of these.

Directions: **For each of the statements below, one or more of the answers is correct. Choose**

   A. If 1, 2, and 3 are correct.
   B. If only 1 and 3 are correct.
   C. If only 2 and 4 are correct.
   D. If only 4 is correct.
   E. If all are correct.

Mood Disorders

13.27 Factors associated with increased mortality among older men include
1. Physical health problems.
2. Retirement.
3. Depression.
4. Change of residence.

13.28 Among elderly patients with a major depressive disorder with onset after age 60
1. 33% relapsed within 12 months.
2. 67% relapsed within 18 months.
3. 55% relapsed within 24 months.
4. Only 7% had a continuous depression.

13.29 Factors complicating the course of depression and its response to treatment include
1. Physical illness.
2. Age.
3. Impaired cognition.
4. Season of the year.

13.30 Factors associated with an improved outcome in late-life depression include
1. Family history of depression.
2. Female sex.
3. Current or recent employment.
4. Absence of substance abuse.

13.31 Seasonal affective disorder may be treated with
1. Lithium carbonate.
2. Carbamazepine.
3. Light therapy.
4. Tricyclic antidepressants.

13.32 Individuals with delusional (psychotic) depression tend
1. To be older.
2. To be male.
3. To respond to ECT.
4. To have little guilt.

13.33 Late-life depression is associated with the following psychological mechanisms
1. Self-reproach.
2. Guilt.
3. Introjection (i.e., the turning inward of hostile feelings toward loss).
4. Loss of self-esteem.

13.34 Retirement and the ending of parenting responsibilities results in changes in
1. Recognition.
2. Self-esteem.
3. Confidence.
4. Sense of mastery.

13.35 Identifiable stressors for older adults associated with an adjustment disorder with depressed mood include
1. Marital problems and difficulty with children.
2. Loss of a social role.
3. Ill-advised change of residence.
4. Retirement.

13.36 Depression has been associated with medical illness with
1. 25% of patients hospitalized with cancer meeting the criteria for a major depressive disorder.
2. 64% of patients with cardiac disease meeting the criteria for a major depressive disorder.
3. 50% of patients with Parkinson's disease meeting the criteria for a major depressive disorder.
4. 28% of patients with vitamin B_{12} (cobalamine) deficiency meeting the criteria for a major depressive disorder.

13.37 Depression presenting as pseudodementia can be distinguished from true dementia by
1. Its rapid onset of cognitive problems.
2. Its relatively short duration of symptoms.
3. A consistent depressed mood associated with cognitive difficulties.
4. A tendency to highlight difficulties.

Mood Disorders

13.38 Late-life schizophrenia may be differentiated from a major depressive illness by
1. A pattern of onset of illness.
2. The presence of psychological distress.
3. Bizarre comments.
4. Poor self-esteem.

13.39 The diagnostic workup of the depressed older person should include
1. History of previous episodes.
2. History of drug or alcohol abuse.
3. Response to previous therapeutic interventions for depressive illness.
4. Family history of depression, suicide, or alcohol abuse.

13.40 Laboratory studies important in the evaluation of the depressed older person include
1. Thyroid panel.
2. Thyroid-stimulating hormone (TSH).
3. Red cell indices.
4. Vitamin B_{12}.

13.41 Contraindications to the use or continued use of tricyclic antidepressants include
1. Second-degree heart block.
2. Bifascicular bundle-branch block.
3. Left bundle-branch block.
4. QT_c interval of 350 milliseconds.

ANSWERS

13.1 The answer is **C**. A community survey of 1,300 older persons living in both urban and rural communities found that only 0.8% were experiencing a current major depressive episode. Some 27% of these elderly community residents reported depressive symptoms, but only 2% had a dysthymic disorder **(p. 236)**.

13.2 The answer is **A**. Among elderly nursing home patients, the rates of major depressive disorder were found to range between 12% to 16% **(p. 237)**.

13.3 The answer is **B.** Some 9.7% of nursing home patients had a diagnosis of bipolar disorder. In a 6-month study of the prevalence of psychiatric disorders in three communities, none of the 3,000 elders interviewed were found to have a current manic episode **(p. 237)**.

13.4 The answer is **B.** The duration of a major depressive episode throughout the life cycle was found to be 9 months **(p. 238)**.

13.5 The answer is **A.** Eighty percent of healthy, depressed elderly treated with combined interpersonal therapy and nortriptyline improved **(p. 238)**.

13.6 The answer is **C.** In a study of treatment-resistant, depressed elderly 15 months after treatment with an antidepressant or ECT, 47% were clinically improved. At 4 years follow-up, 71% were improved **(pp. 238–239)**.

13.7 The answer is **D.** The DST was not found to be of value in predicting long-term follow-up. Data from metaanalysis of 144 studies concluded that nonsuppression of cortisol on baseline DST does predict a poorer response to placebo. Persistent suppression on DST after treatment is associated with a high risk of early relapse and poor outcome after discharge. Baseline DST status does not predict response to antidepressant treatment or outcome after hospital discharge **(p. 239)**.

13.8 The answer is **A.** Depressed patients who reported an adequate social support network at the time of the index episode were 2.3 times more likely (44% versus 19%) to have recovered than depressed patients who reported an impaired social network **(p. 239)**.

13.9 The answer is **D.** Organic insults (stroke, head trauma, other brain insults) increased cerebral vulnerability and played a stronger role than life events in precipitating late-onset mania **(p. 240)**.

13.10 The answer is **B.** Studies of elderly patients with unipolar depression suggest that the genetic contribution is weaker in late-life depression than observed at earlier stages of the life cycle **(p. 240)**.

13.11 The answer is **A.** Although numerous neurotransmitters and neuroendocrine changes are common to old age and depressive illness, the prevalence of depression and bipolar disorder in late life is relatively low. The data suggest that older persons are not uniquely predisposed to depression **(p. 241)**.

Mood Disorders

13.12 The answer is **D**. Elderly patients with bipolar disorder may exhibit an elevated or irritable mood or a depressive admixture with manic symptomatology **(p. 242)**.

13.13 The answer is **E**. Elderly African-American men in particular may conceal or deny symptoms of depression on self-report **(p. 243)**.

13.14 The answer is **C**. Criteria for a diagnosis of depression not otherwise specified requires the presence of symptoms for less than 2 weeks. If dysphoric symptoms are present for 2 weeks, the criteria for major depressive disorder may be met **(p. 244)**.

13.15 The answer is **D**. Somatic symptoms of distress associated with bereavement include tightness in the throat, shortness of breath, sighing respirations, lassitude, and loss of appetite **(p. 244)**.

13.16 The answer is **D**. Medications are the most common toxic cause of substance-induced mood disorders. Medications that can precipitate depressive symptoms include beta-blockers, benzodiazepines, clonidine, methyldopa, and reserpine **(p. 245)**.

13.17 The answer is **A**. Some 25% of patients with hypochondriacal symptoms attempted suicide **(p. 250)**.

13.18 The answer is **C**. The diagnosis of depression should not be made until the patient is sober for at least 2 weeks. Alcohol withdrawal may include dysphoria and other depressive symptoms **(p. 250)**.

13.19 The answer is **C**. Cognitive behavioral therapy is the only psychotherapy developed specifically to treat depression. Its advantage in the elderly is that it is directive and time limited, requiring 10–25 sessions to complete **(p. 253)**.

13.20 The answer is **A**. A nortriptyline dose of 25–50 mg at bedtime is frequently sufficient to relieve depressive symptoms **(p. 254)**.

13.21 The answer is **C**. An interval of 1–2 weeks must elapse between stopping an SSRI and starting an MAOI in order to avoid a serotonergic syndrome. In the case of stopping fluoxetine with its long-acting active metabolite (norfluoxetine), an interval of 2–4 weeks is indicated **(p. 254)**.

13.22 The answer is **B**. Before the initiation of ECT, an MAOI should be withdrawn for 10–14 days before the first treatment to prevent toxic interactions or effects of the MAOI with the anesthetic used for ECT **(p. 255)**.

13.23 The answer is **C**. To achieve optimal results, the seizure induced with ECT should last 25 seconds **(p. 255)**.

13.24 The answer is **A**. When ECT is used in depressed patients who were nonresponders to antidepressant medication, the response rate is usually 80% or greater **(p. 256)**.

13.25 The answer is **D**. When the efficacy of ECT in elderly depressed patients with dementia was studied, a response rate of 86% was found. Only 21% of these patients experienced a significant worsening of cognition, with the cognitive problem being transient. Forty-nine percent of patients treated with ECT showed improvement in memory function after treatment **(p. 256)**.

13.26 The answer is **D**. Family members can assist in the evaluation of the older depressed patients by observing changes in behavior such as increased withdrawal, decreased verbalization, and preoccupation with medication or weapons. The family can assist by removing possible implements of suicide from easy access. When depressive symptoms become so severe that hospitalization is required, family members are valuable in facilitating hospitalization **(p. 257)**.

13.27 The answer is **B**. Mortality among depressed men was found to be three times the expected rate. After separating the sample by health status, older men with increased mortality had physical health problems and depression **(p. 238)**.

13.28 The answer is **D**. In a study of 100 elderly psychiatric patients with severe major depressive disorder followed for 3–8 years, only 7% had continuous depression. Of these patients 60% remained well throughout the follow-up or had relapses with complete recovery **(p. 238)**.

13.29 The answer is **B**. Physical illness and impaired cognitive function are factors that may complicate the course of depression and response to treatment of the depressive illness **(p. 239)**.

13.30 The answer is **E**. Factors associated with an improved outcome in late-life depression included a history of recovery from previous episodes, family history of depression, female sex, extroverted personality, current or recent employment, absence of substance abuse, no history of major psychiatric disorder, less severe depressive symptomatology, and absence of major life events **(p. 239)**.

Mood Disorders 77

13.31 The answer is **A.** Lithium carbonate, or carbamazepine, and light therapy (using high-intensity light) have been shown to be effective in the treatment of seasonal affective disorder. The use of TCAs may perpetuate seasonal affective disorder and should not be used because they increase the likelihood of rapid cycling **(p. 243)**.

13.32 The answer is **B.** Individuals with delusional depression are more likely to be older and to respond to ECT rather than tricyclic antidepressants. Guilt may predominate the delusional picture and involve a trivial episode that occurred many years before the onset of depression **(p. 243)**.

13.33 The answer is **D.** Late-life depression is associated the loss of self-esteem that results from multiple factors: the older person's inability to supply needs and drives and to defend against threats to the older person's security. The classic psychological mechanisms of dysthymia—self-reproach, guilt, and the turning inward of hostile feelings toward loss (introjection)—are not seen in late-life dysthymic disorder **(p. 243)**.

13.34 The answer is **B.** Recognition, self-esteem, and confidence are affected in the elderly. Retirement and the ending of the parenting role decrease the means and opportunity to meet these needs **(p. 244)**.

13.35 The answer is **A.** Identifiable stressors for the elderly associated with an adjustment disorder with depressed mood include marital problems, difficulty with children, loss of social role, and an ill-advised change in residence. Retirement is not a source of excessive stress for the elderly **(p. 245)**.

13.36 The answer is **E.** Depression has been associated with medical illnesses, including cardiovascular disease, endocrine disturbances, Parkinson's disease, stroke, diabetes, cancer, chronic pain, chronic fatigue syndrome, and fibromyalgia **(p. 245)**. Various studies have found that 25% of patients hospitalized for cancer meet criteria for depression; 64% of patients with cardiac disease, 50% of patients with Parkinson's disease, and 28% of patients with vitamin B_{12} (cobalamin) deficiency reported depressive symptoms **(pp. 246–247)**.

13.37 The answer is **E.** Depressed patients with cognitive difficulties not caused by true dementia are more likely to respond with "I don't know" on the mental status examination. The pseudodementia of depression can be differentiated from true dementia by the rapid onset of cognitive problems, the relative short duration of symptoms, a consistent depressed mood associated with cognitive difficulties, and a tendency to highlight difficulties **(p. 248)**.

13.38 The answer is **A**. Late-life schizophrenia can be differentiated from a major depressive illness by a history of gradual onset of illness, gradual withdrawal, bizarre comments, and elaborate preparations for safety. Paranoid elders rarely have poor self-esteem but are distressed and focus all of their difficulties on a hostile environment **(p. 249)**.

13.39 The answer is **E**. The evaluation of the depressed older person should include an assessment of the duration of the current depressive episode. Important historical information includes a history of previous episodes; a history of drug or alcohol abuse; the history of response to previous therapeutic interventions for depressive illness; and a family history of depression, suicide, and/or alcohol abuse **(p. 250)**.

13.40 The answer is **E**. Thyroid panel with TSH, red cell indices, and vitamin B_{12} are important laboratory studies to rule out hypothyroidism, anemia, and vitamin B_{12} deficiency as the etiology of the depressive symptoms **(p. 251)**.

13.41 The answer is **A**. An ECG should be obtained before treatment and again after therapeutic blood levels have been achieved. Treatment with TCAs should not be initiated or should be withdrawn if the ECG shows a second-degree heart block or higher, a bifascicular bundle-branch block, a left bundle-branch block, or a QT_c interval of greater than 480 milliseconds **(p. 254)**.

CHAPTER 14

Schizophrenia and Paranoid Disorders

QUESTIONS

Directions: **Select the single best response for each of the following questions.**

14.1 The DSM-III criteria for a diagnosis of schizophrenia required

   A. The presence of a fixed delusion.
   B. The presence of command hallucinations.
   C. An onset before age 45.
   D. All of these.
   E. None of these.

14.2 The differential diagnosis of schizophrenia-like symptoms in late life includes

   A. Suspiciousness.
   B. Transitional paranoid reactions.
   C. Paraphrenia.
   D. All of these.
   E. None of these.

14.3 Data from the Duke University Epidemiology Catchment Area (ECA) survey site of persons age 60 and older found an unweighted prevalence of schizophrenia of

   A. 1.0%.
   B. 0.2%.
   C. 2.0%.
   D. All of these.
   E. None of these.

14.4 Organic factors that can cause paranoid or schizophrenia-like symptoms include
   A. Niacin deficiency.
   B. Parathyroid disorder.
   C. Multiple sclerosis.
   D. All of these.
   E. None of these.

14.5 The transitional paranoid reaction may be seen in persons who
   A. Have severe primary degenerative dementia.
   B. Have multiinfarct dementia.
   C. Live in long-term care facilities.
   D. All of these.
   E. None of these.

14.6 The most important and frequent cause of paranoid symptoms in the elderly is
   A. Delirium.
   B. Dementia.
   C. Schizophrenia.
   D. All of these.
   E. None of these.

14.7 Women are more likely to be diagnosed with paraphrenia than men. The female-to-male ratio is
   A. 3:1.
   B. 5:1.
   C. 10:1.
   D. All of these.
   E. None of these.

14.8 In treating the older patient with paranoid symptoms or paraphrenia, the dose of thioridazine must be adjusted to avoid falls due to orthostatic hypotension and to prevent outflow obstruction in men with benign prostatic hypertrophy. The initial total daily dose should be
   A. Below 80 mg.
   B. Below 60 mg.
   C. Below 40 mg.
   D. All of these.
   E. None of these.

Schizophrenia and Paranoid Disorders

Directions: For each of the statements below, one or more of the answers is correct. Choose

- A. If 1, 2, and 3 are correct.
- B. If only 1 and 3 are correct.
- C. If only 2 and 4 are correct.
- D. If only 4 is correct.
- E. If all are correct.

14.9 Roth defined late *paraphrenia* to describe a syndrome characterized by
1. Onset of symptoms after age 60.
2. Symptoms occurring in a well personality with affective response intact.
3. A well-organized system of paranoid delusions.
4. An outcome different from schizophrenia patients with affective disorders or dementia.

14.10 Factors contributing to suspiciousness in the elderly include
1. Loss of memory and attention.
2. Hearing deficits.
3. Visual deficits.
4. Residence in a long-term care facility.

14.11 Transitional paranoid reaction is seen in
1. Women who live alone.
2. Men who live alone.
3. Women who believe a plot exists against them.
4. Men who believe a plot exists against them.

14.12 Patients with schizophrenia and paraphrenia both have
1. Disturbance of affect.
2. Disturbance of volition.
3. Disturbance in function.
4. Paranoid delusions and hallucinations.

14.13 Late-onset schizophrenia is characterized by
1. Bizarre delusions (often persecutory in nature).
2. Auditory hallucinations.
3. Less common thought broadcasting and thought insertion.
4. A more benign course than early-onset schizophrenia.

14.14 The elderly patient with delirium compared with a younger patient with delirium
   1. Is more likely to report hallucinations associated with delusional thinking.
   2. Is less likely to report hallucinations associated with delusional thinking.
   3. Is more likely to report suspiciousness.
   4. Exhibits impoverished and incoherent thought processes and impaired reasoning.

14.15 Treatment of the older patient with paranoid or schizophrenic syndromes should include
   1. Antipsychotic medication to help sleep and anxiety.
   2. A trusting supportive relationship with a clinician.
   3. The development of a network of community contacts.
   4. Direct confrontation of the paranoid ideation.

14.16 Risk factors for the development of late-onset paraphrenia include
   1. Being female gender and having been married.
   2. Being socially isolated due to the loss of family and friends.
   3. Having sensory impairment.
   4. Having a schizophrenic sibling.

ANSWERS

14.1 The answer is **C**. The DSM-III criteria requirement of onset of symptoms before age 45 for a diagnosis of schizophrenia was very controversial and was revised in DSM-III-R to include a late-onset criteria for the development of symptoms of schizophrenia after age 44. In DSM-IV there is no age criterion, and the late-onset diagnostic category has been deleted **(p. 266)**.

14.2 The answer is **D**. The differential diagnosis of schizophrenia-like symptoms with an onset in late life should include suspiciousness, transitional paranoid reactions, and paraphrenia **(pp. 267–268)**.

14.3 The answer is **B**. Among the 1,600 individuals age 60 and older studied by Duke University at the ECA site in Durham, North Carolina, an unweighted prevalence rate of 0.2% was found for schizophrenia or

Schizophrenia and Paranoid Disorders 83

schizophreniform disorder. Eight percent of the sample reported at least one current symptom of schizophrenia, 4.3% reported delusions, and 5.4% reported hallucinations **(p. 265)**.

14.4 The answer is **D**. Paranoid or schizophrenia-like symptoms may be caused by medical conditions (thyroid, parathyroid, adrenal, and pancreatic dysfunction), neurologic conditions (all varieties of dementia seizure disorders, hydrocephalus, multiple sclerosis, brain tumors, neurosyphilis), vitamin deficiencies (B_{12}, thiamine, niacin, folote), and other disorders **(p. 269)**.

14.5 The answer is **D**. Patients with severe dementia, either primary degenerative or multiinfarct, and patients who live in long-term care facilities can exhibit transitional paranoid reactions **(p. 267)**.

14.6 The answer is **A**. Transient cognitive disturbance (e.g., delirium) is the most frequent cause of paranoid symptoms in the elderly **(p. 270)**.

14.7 The answer is **B**. The female-to-male ratio in patients with paraphrenia is 5:1 in contrast to a sex ratio of 1:1 in patients with schizophrenia **(p. 271)**.

14.8 The answer is **A**. To avoid the complications of orthostatic hypotension and outflow obstruction caused by the anticholinergic side effects of thioridazine, the total daily dose should be less than 80 mg **(p. 273)**.

14.9 The answer is **E**. Roth introduced the term *paraphrenia* to describe patients with these characteristics. The term *late paraphrenia* was developed to describe this syndrome that resembled schizophrenia and occurred frequently among the elderly **(p. 266)**.

14.10 The answer is **E**. Older persons with memory impairment and deficits in hearing or vision report suspiciousness because of their limited ability to interpret their environment as well as a sense of loss of control. For persons with dementing illness in long-term care facilities, suspiciousness may manifest as accusation against family and staff that are disjointed and not focused **(p. 267)**.

14.11 The answer is **B**. Women living alone who believe that a plot exists against them most frequently exhibit the focal, narrow, situational paranoid hallucinations that characterize the transitional paranoid reaction **(p. 267)**.

14.12 The answer is **D**. The syndrome of late-onset schizophrenia is identified as a primary disorder not caused by either affective illness or an organic mental disorder. The disturbances of volition and function seen in patients with schizophrenia are not prominent. Paranoid delusions and hallucinations are seen in both schizophrenia and paraphrenia **(p. 268)**.

14.13 The answer is **E.** Late-onset schizophrenia is characterized by bizarre delusions (often persecutory in nature) and auditory hallucinations. Thought broadcasting and thought insertion are less common among the elderly patient with late-onset schizophrenia, and the course of illness for these patients is more benign **(p. 268)**.

14.14 The answer is **C.** In contrast to younger patients with delirium, the older patient with delirium is less likely to report florid hallucinations associated with delusional thinking. Impoverishment and incoherence of thought processes with impaired reasoning and judgment are associated with generalized suspiciousness **(p. 271)**.

14.15 The answer is **A.** Older, paranoid patients are willing to take medication with an explanation that the medication will improve sleep and decrease anxiety. The establishment of a trusting, supportive relationship with a clinician will assist the older person in interpretation of his or her environment. The development of a relationship with people in the patient's social network is important. Direct confrontation of a fixed, false belief is nonproductive and may result in the patient leaving treatment **(p. 274)**.

14.16 The answer is **E.** All are characteristics of patients with late-onset schizophrenia. The expectancy rate for schizophrenia in the first-degree relatives of patients with late-onset schizophrenia of 2.5% is less than the 10% rate reported among the siblings of patients with early-onset schizophrenia **(p. 272)**.

CHAPTER 15

Anxiety and Panic Disorders

QUESTIONS

Directions: **Select the single best response for each of the following questions.**

15.1 *Anxiety disorders* may be best defined as being composed of
   A. Depression.
   B. Worry and fearfulness.
   C. Morbid anxiety.
   D. Palpitations.
   E. None of these.

15.2 *Panic attacks* are best defined as
   A. Tingling in hands and feet and shortness of breath.
   B. Recurrent episodes of severe anxiety or fear.
   C. Fear of dying or hot and cold flashes.
   D. All of these.
   E. None of these.

15.3 A characteristic of late-onset panic disorders (LOPD) is
   A. Greater score on somatization measures.
   B. Fewer panic symptoms.
   C. Greater avoidance.
   D. All of these.
   E. None of these.

15.4 Depression is most frequently seen with
   A. Specific phobia.
   B. Generalized anxiety disorder.
   C. Acute stress disorder.
   D. All of these.
   E. None of these.

15.5 When starting a pharmacological management of anxiety, one should
   A. "Start low and go slow."
   B. Obtain laboratory studies to assess thyroid function and liver function.
   C. Titrate the dose upward rapidly.
   D. All of these.
   E. None of these.

15.6 A medication helpful in the management of severe anxiety and agitation associated with dementia is
   A. Trazodone.
   B. Phenelzine.
   C. Fluoxetine.
   D. All of these.
   E. None of these.

Directions: **For each of the statements below, one or more of the answers is correct. Choose**

   A. If 1, 2, and 3 are correct.
   B. If only 1 and 3 are correct.
   C. If only 2 and 4 are correct.
   D. If only 4 is correct.
   E. If all are correct.

15.7 Older persons may have a persistent fear of social situations such as
   1. Eating in public.
   2. Speaking in public.
   3. Writing in public.
   4. All of these.

15.8 Specific anxiety and panic disorders that have been studied in the elderly include
   1. Agoraphobia without a history of panic disorders.
   2. Specific phobia.
   3. Acute stress disorder.
   4. Obsessive-compulsive disorder.

15.9 Specific factors affecting the diagnosis of anxiety include
1. Medical illness.
2. Over-the-counter medications.
3. Sedative-hypnotic or alcohol withdrawal.
4. Depression.

15.10 Nonselective beta-blockers (β_2 and β_2) (e.g., propranolol and pindolol) should be used with caution in medically ill elderly patients with
1. Chronic obstructive pulmonary disease.
2. Diabetes mellitus.
3. Congestive heart failure.
4. Hypotension.

ANSWERS

15.1 The answer is **C**. Anxiety disorders comprised the various signs and symptoms of morbid, unjustifiably excessive anxiety manifested by worry, fearfulness, phobias, palpitations, and hyperventilation **(p. 279)**.

15.2 The answer is **B**. Panic attacks, the recurrent episodes of severe anxiety and fear, comprise panic disorder. Various somatic symptoms (tingling of the hands and feet, shortness of breath) as well as cognitive symptoms (fear of dying or losing control) are experienced by the patient with panic disorder **(p. 280)**.

15.3 The answer is **B**. Patients with LOPD compared with patients with early-onset panic disorder were found to have fewer panic symptoms, less avoidance, and lower scores on somatization measures **(p. 280)**.

15.4 The answer is **B**. Older patients with generalized anxiety disorder may present with symptoms of depression, making the therapist's decision about diagnosis and treatment difficult **(p. 281)**.

15.5 The answer is **A**. In the elderly, the normal physiologic changes of aging can affect the distribution of medication and their metabolism. It is important to prevent the accumulation of medication by prescribing lower doses in the early stages of treatment and by slowly increasing the dosage **(p. 284)**.

15.6 The answer is **A**. Trazodone, a selective serotonin reuptake inhibitor antidepressant, has been shown to be useful in the management of severe anxiety and agitation associated with dementia **(p. 285)**.

15.7 The answer is **B**. Because of the use of dentures and the presence of tremors in the elderly, phobias involving these social situations more than public speaking are of concern in the elderly **(p. 280)**.

15.8 The answer is **D**. Systematic studies of agoraphobia without history of panic disorder and specific phobia have not been completed in the elderly, and acute stress disorder is a new diagnostic category in DSM-IV **(pp. 280–281)**. Epidemiologic studies of the elderly report a 6-month prevalence rate of obsessive-compulsive disorder of 1.5% **(p. 281)**.

15.9 The answer is **E**. Medical illness, over-the-counter and prescribed medication, withdrawal from sedative hypnotics or alcohol, and depression can produce symptoms of anxiety **(pp. 282–283)**.

15.10 The answer is **A**. Although useful for some elderly patients with agitation and anxiety and in patients with dementia and extreme agitation, nonselective β_1 and β_2 beta-blockers (propranolol and pindolol) should be used with caution in medically ill elderly patients. Specific diseases of concern include chronic obstructive pulmonary disease, diabetes mellitus, and congestive cardiac failure **(p. 285)**.

CHAPTER 16

Somatoform and Psychosexual Disorders

QUESTIONS

Directions: **Select the single best response for each of the following questions.**

16.1 The term *hypochondriasis* is based on the Greek term *hypochondrium,* which refers to

   A. The part of the body between the umbilicus and the eschusheon.
   B. The part of the body between the ribs and the xiphoid cartilage.
   C. The part of the body between the clavicals and the xiphoid cartilage.
   D. All of these.
   E. None of these.

16.2 The diagnosis of hypochondriasis in the elderly is complicated by

   A. The existence of physical disabilities.
   B. The presence of disease.
   C. The socioeconomic stressors associated with aging.
   D. All of these.
   E. None of these.

16.3 *Hypochondriasis* is defined as

   A. An anxious preoccupation with the body or a portion of the body that is believed to be diseased or functioning improperly.
   B. A persistent preoccupation with the possibility of having a progressive physical disorder associated with marked depression and anxiety.
   C. A delusional belief that one has a serious disease based on the person's misinterpretation of bodily symptoms.
   D. All of these.
   E. None of these.

16.4 The Duke Longitudinal Study of Aging used "high bodily concern" as a measure of hypochondriasis. These data found that over a 20-year period, hypochondriasis was

A. Fixed and persistent.
B. Transient.
C. Episodic.
D. All of these.
E. None of these.

16.5 Treatment of hypochondriasis in the elderly must recognize

A. That hypochondriasis in this population is a biological/psychosocial phenomenon.
B. That many of these patients respond favorably to a combined medical-psychotherapeutic approach.
C. That it is possible for true organic illness to develop or coexist with hypochondriasis.
D. All of these.
E. None of these.

16.6 Hypochondriasis is associated with

A. Psychosis.
B. Anxiety.
C. Depression.
D. All of these.
E. None of these.

16.7 Elderly persons in the Duke Longitudinal Study with hypochondriasis ("high bodily concern")

A. Sought medical attention frequently.
B. Took prescribed medication faithfully.
C. Responded to the suggestions of family and friends.
D. All of these.
E. None of these.

16.8 Psychological defense mechanisms that play a role in the dynamics of hypochondriasis are reinforced by

A. Health professionals.
B. Family members.
C. Secondary gain.
D. All of these.
E. None of these.

Somatoform and Psychosexual Disorders

16.9 Psychological defense mechanisms important in the role of hypochondriasis include
   A. Symptoms as an explanation of failure.
   B. Withdrawal of interest from others and a redirection of psychic interest to the body and its functions.
   C. Shifting anxiety from a specific psychic conflict to a less threatening body function.
   D. All of these.
   E. None of these.

16.10 The hypochondriacal patient should be seen
   A. Daily.
   B. Weekly.
   C. Twice a week.
   D. All of these.
   E. None of these.

16.11 Persistent pain is
   A. Seen more frequently in late middle life.
   B. Afflicts 25%–50% of community-resident elderly.
   C. Is usually associated with degenerative conditions.
   D. All of these.
   E. None of these.

16.12 Chronic pain seen in younger adults is due to
   A. Arthralgia.
   B. Pleuritic pain.
   C. Headaches and backaches.
   D. All of these.
   E. None of these.

16.13 Approaches to the relief of pain have included
   A. Extracts of white poppy.
   B. Acupuncture.
   C. Transcutaneous electrical nerve stimulation (TENS).
   D. All of these.
   E. None of these.

16.14 The psychopathology of the paraphilias involves
   A. A distortion of the sex object.
   B. An aberration of sexual expression.
   C. An aberration of sexual enjoyment.
   D. All of these.
   E. None of these.

16.15 Sexual dysfunctions are
   A. Psychological disturbances.
   B. Linked to mental and emotional disorder.
   C. Seen only in late life.
   D. All of these.
   E. None of these.

16.16 The most important change in male sexual function associated with aging is
   A. An increase in the frequency of ejaculation and the need to ejaculate.
   B. A decrease in the frequency of ejaculation and the need to ejaculate.
   C. An increase in the frequency of ejaculation and a decrease in the need to ejaculate.
   D. All of these.
   E. None of these.

16.17 The physiological counterpart of male erection is
   A. Vaginal lubrication.
   B. Clitoral erection.
   C. Labial engorgement.
   D. All of these.
   E. None of these.

16.18 Estrogen replacement is important in older women. Without exogenous sources,
   A. Vaginal mucosal lining becomes very thin.
   B. Vaginal mucosal lining becomes atrophic.
   C. Local irritation and bleeding can result from the trauma of intercourse.
   D. None of these.
   E. All of these.

Somatoform and Psychosexual Disorders 93

16.19 A uterine spasm associated with orgasm in postmenopausal women may be experienced as severe lower abdominal pain, which reflects
   A. Uterine atrophy.
   B. A state of deconditioning of the abdominal muscles.
   C. A state of sex steroid starvation.
   D. All of these.
   E. None of these.

16.20 Marriage trends identified among older persons include
   A. 67% of older men versus 33% of older women live with a spouse.
   B. Among persons age 75 and older, twice as many men as women are married.
   C. 37% of brides age 65 and older are marrying younger men.
   D. All of these.
   E. None of these.

16.21 The most common cause of impotence in older males is
   A. Vascular disease involving the penile arteries.
   B. Diabetes.
   C. Psychological origin.
   D. All of these.
   E. None of these.

16.22 Men
   A. May ejaculate with a flaccid penis.
   B. Can experience an orgasm without an erection.
   C. Have different neuronal mechanisms that control erection, arousal, and ejaculation.
   D. All of these.
   E. None of these.

16.23 Older gay men
   A. Were observed to be much more youth oriented than heterosexual males.
   B. Tended to view aging more negatively.
   C. Tended to view themselves as "old" at earlier ages.
   D. All of these.
   E. None of these.

16.24 Sexual intimacy is an unfavorable experience when it is
- A. Devoid of mutual caring.
- B. Devoid of responsibility.
- C. Devoid of open communication.
- D. All of these.
- E. None of these.

Directions: **For each of the statements below, one or more of the answers is correct. Choose**

- **A. If 1, 2, and 3 are correct.**
- **B. If only 1 and 3 are correct.**
- **C. If only 2 and 4 are correct.**
- **D. If only 4 is correct.**
- **E. If all are correct.**

16.25 The ancient Greeks believed that the hypochondrium was the seat of
1. Morbid anxiety associated with oneself.
2. Depression or bad mood.
3. Simulated disease.
4. Psychosis.

16.26 Older persons participating in the Duke Longitudinal Studies who developed high bodily concern (hypochondriasis) were found
1. To have a history of other psychoneurotic reactions.
2. To have a much lower evaluation of life satisfaction.
3. To have fewer friends.
4. To have fewer wholesome attitudes toward their friends.

16.27 Disorders that overlap or are seen frequently with hypochondriasis include
1. Depressive disorders.
2. Anxiety disorders.
3. Somatoform disorders.
4. Psychotic disorders.

16.28 Predisposing factors to the development of hypochondriasis identified by Lipowski included
1. Genetics.
2. Developmental learning.
3. Personality.
4. Sociocultural environment.

Somatoform and Psychosexual Disorders

16.29 Theories of hypochondriasis as a learned behavior from childhood suggest that
1. Children with "physical" disorders get anxious attention from their parents.
2. Children with mental disorders get anxious attention from parents.
3. Children learn that being sick allows them to avoid unpleasant duties.
4. Children learn that being sick does not affect homework.

16.30 Factors contributing to the development of hypochondriasis in elderly patients include
1. Recurrent exposure to criticism in a situation without the possibility of escape.
2. Reduction in economic status and isolation due to socioeconomic factors.
3. Loss of spouse and friends.
4. Deterioration in marital satisfaction.

16.31 Treatment techniques of the hypochondriacal patient should include
1. A supportive statement and manner.
2. A false diagnosis.
3. Avoidance of statements that threaten the patient's hypochondriacal defense.
4. Utilization of placebo medication.

16.32 Psychiatrists working with elderly hypochondriacal patients may encounter
1. Resistance.
2. Hostility.
3. Confrontation.
4. Violence.

16.33 Older patients may experience
1. Painless myocardial infarction.
2. The absence of fever and leukocytosis with appendicitis.
3. Persistent pain with osteoarthritis.
4. A change in pain threshold for noxious stimuli.

16.34 Chronic pain cannot be completely eliminated in the elderly. A more realistic goal is
1. To reduce the intensity of pain exacerbations.
2. To reduce the frequency of pain exacerbations.
3. To restore functional capacity.
4. To improve mood and the quality of life.

16.35 Hormone (testosterone) replacement in the older man is of concern because
1. Testosterone frequently exacerbates benign prostatic hypertrophy (BPH).
2. Testosterone is contraindicated if prostatic carcinoma is suspected.
3. Testosterone may produce polycythemia.
4. Testosterone will improve prostate lubrication.

16.36 The continuation of sexual activity in late life is dependent on
1. The availability of a sexual partner.
2. The physical and mental health of the partners.
3. The pattern of sexual interest and activity established in early adulthood.
4. Age under 65.

16.37 Painful sexual intercourse in older women can be due to
1. Changes in diet.
2. Estrogen deficiency.
3. Decreased activity.
4. A diseased, retroverted uterus.

16.38 Sexual behavioral problems among nursing home residents are affected by
1. The paternalistic attitudes of staff.
2. The negative attitude of staff concerning older patients being sexually active.
3. The staff's perception of the nursing home resident as a victim and a perpetrator.
4. The elderly resident's interests and attitudes toward sexuality in the past.

Somatoform and Psychosexual Disorders

ANSWERS

16.1 The answer is **B**. In the ancient Greek language, the *hypochondrium* referred to the part of the body between the ribs and the xiphoid cartilage **(p. 291)**.

16.2 The answer is **D**. Factors complicating the diagnosis of hypochondriasis in the elderly include the existence of physical disabilities, the presence of disease, and the socioeconomic stressors (retirement, moving, death of family and friends) that are age related **(p. 292)**.

16.3 The answer is **A**. In this text, *hypochondriasis* is defined by DSM-IV criteria as "a disorder that is an anxious preoccupation with the body or part of the body that is believed to be diseased or functioning improperly." Although the ICD-10 criteria for hypochondriasis disorder include "marked depression and anxiety" as part of the definition of the disorder, these are not part of the DSM-IV criteria. By the DSM-IV diagnostic criteria for hypochondriasis, the presence of a delusional belief rules out the diagnosis of hypochondriasis and suggests either a delusional disorder somatic type or body dysmorphic disorder **(pp. 291–292)**.

16.4 The answer is **B**. Data from the Duke Longitudinal Study of Aging found that transient hypochondriasis was common in a general medical clinic **(pp. 292, 295)**.

16.5 The answer is **D**. In the elderly, hypochondriasis is frequently a biological/psychosocial phenomenon, and a combined medical-psychotherapeutic approach produces a favorable response. Remaining alert to the possibility of the coexistence or development of a true organic illness is important in this population **(pp. 292–293)**.

16.6 The answer is **C**. Hypochondriacal symptoms may be associated with overt symptoms of anxiety or depression. In one study of 152 depressed patients over age 60, 66% of men and 62% of women reported hypochondriacal symptoms. The most common symptom was constipation **(p. 293)**.

16.7 The answer is **E**. Elderly persons with "high bodily concern" in the Duke Longitudinal Study resisted the urging of family and friends to seek medical treatment for their multiple symptoms. Many used home remedies and excessively used over-the-counter medication. If forced by family and friends to seek medical treatment, their pattern of maintaining social adjustment and self-esteem was threatened, and the hypochondriacal pattern sometimes became solidified **(p. 295)**.

16.8 The answer is **C**. The psychological defense mechanisms involved in the dynamics of hypochondriasis are reinforced by secondary gain. *Secondary gain* is a term describing the increased attention and sympathy from friends and health care providers originally generated by the symptoms **(p. 295)**.

16.9 The answer is **D**. Four psychological defense mechanisms have been identified as playing an important role in the dynamics of hypochondriasis in the elderly: 1) the symptoms may be used as an explanation for failure to meet personal and social expectations and to avoid or excuse recurrent failure; 2) experiencing increasing isolation, the patient may withdraw psychic interest from other persons or objects and redirect it to the self, the body, and bodily functions; 3) the patient may shift anxiety from a specific psychiatric conflict to a less-threatening bodily function; 4) the symptoms may be a means of self-punishment and atonement for unacceptable hostile feelings toward persons close to the individual **(p. 295)**.

16.10 The answer is **B**. It is best to see the hypochondriacal patient once a week for the initial 8–10 weeks of treatment at a definite time. The clinician should expect that the hypochondriacal patient will reject the initial appointment time as inconvenient. This behavior has been identified as a way of testing the physician to determine the extent of his or her interest in the patient **(pp. 297–298)**. After the initial interview, which may be 90 minutes, return visits should be 15–20 minutes **(p. 298)**.

16.11 The answer is **D**. Persistent pain is seen more frequently in late and older middle life. It affects 25%–50% of community-resident elderly and is associated with degenerative conditions, pathological conditions (cancer), and trauma to the body and the brain **(p. 299)**.

16.12 The answer is **D**. Persistent or frequently recurring pain (chronic pain) in younger adults is produced by arthralgia, pleuritic pain, headaches, and backaches **(p. 300)**.

16.13 The answer is **D**. Different cultures at different times have identified approaches to the treatment of pain. Ancient Egyptians used the extract from the white poppy to relieve pain, as well as electric fish found in the Nile River. The use of fish bones, stones, and bamboo sticks to stimulate tissue at special sites to relieve pain (textbook of Oriental medicine, *Nei*

Somatoform and Psychosexual Disorders 99

Ching) evolved in 1955 to the technique of acupuncture anesthesia. Sweden derived the TENS technique for pain control from acupuncture **(p. 301)**.

16.14 The answer is **D**. Paraphilic disorders involve a distortion of the sex object and an aberration of sexual expression and enjoyment **(p. 302)**.

16.15 The answer is **B**. Sexual dysfunctions are manifested by physiological disturbances linked to mental and emotional disorders **(p. 302)**.

16.16 The answer is **B**. A reduction in the frequency of ejaculation and a reduction in the need to ejaculate are the most important age-associated changes in male sexual function **(p. 303)**.

16.17 The answer is **A**. The production of vaginal lubrication is the exact physiological counterpart of male erection **(p. 304)**.

16.18 The answer is **D**. Without estrogen replacement in older, postmenopausal women, the vaginal mucosal lining becomes very thin and atrophic. The trauma associated with intercourse can result in local irritation and bleeding **(p. 304)**.

16.19 The answer is **C**. In younger women, the uterus contracts rhythmically with orgasm in a pattern similar to the contractions of the first stage of labor. With advancing years, the rhythm of the contractions may be lost. A spasm can occur and may be experienced as severe lower abdominal pain in the postmenopausal woman. This type of spastic uterine response accompanying orgasm reflects a state of sex steroid starvation **(p. 304)**.

16.20 The answer is **D**. Although most older men are married, most older women are widows. There are four times as many widows as widowers. Two-thirds of men age 65 and older live with wives in contrast to only one-third of women living with husbands. Among persons age 75, and older twice as many men compared with women are married to spouses under age 75. One study reported that 37.1% of brides age 65 years and older were marrying younger men **(p. 305)**.

16.21 The answer is **A**. The most common cause of impotence in older males is vascular disease involving the penile arteries. In a sample of 136 patients treated for impotence, 61% were impotent due to vascular pathology, 18% were impotent due to diabetes, and 15% were impotent due to psychological factors **(p. 306)**.

16.22 The answer is **D**. With aging, there is a diminution in the volume of the ejaculate as well as the force with which the ejaculate is expelled. Men are capable of ejaculating without an erection and can experience an orgasm with a flaccid penis. This is usually the result of anxiety. This can be explained on the basis of different neuronal mechanisms controlling erection, arousal, and ejaculation **(p. 306)**.

16.23 The answer is **D**. Older gay men were found to be more youth oriented and tended to view aging more negatively than heterosexual males. Homosexual men tended to consider themselves "old" at earlier ages than did heterosexual men **(p. 307)**.

16.24 The answer is **D**. Intimacy has been said to occur "when people delight each other and delight in each other in an atmosphere of security based upon mutuality, reciprocity, and total trust in each other." Sexual behavior is one type of intimacy. It is an unfavorable experience if it is devoid of mutual caring, responsibility, and open communication **(p. 307)**.

16.25 The answer is **A**. The hypochondrium was identified by the ancient Greeks as the seat of morbid anxiety associated with oneself, depression, bad mood, or simulated disease. Although the theory of the spleen as the seat of morbid anxiety has not endured, the term *hypochondriasis* has survived **(p. 291)**.

16.26 The answer is **E**. Data from the Duke Longitudinal Studies over a 20-year period found that older persons with "high bodily concern" initially or who later developed it have specific characteristics. These older persons were found "to have a history of other psychoneurotic reaction, to have a much lower evaluation of life satisfactions, to have fewer friends, and to have fewer wholesome attitudes toward their friends **(p. 292)**."

16.27 The answer is **A**. A review of patient histories has shown a considerable overlap between symptoms of hypochondriasis and the manifestations of depression and anxiety disorders. The considerable overlap between hypochondriasis and somatization disorder led investigators to conclude that these two diagnostic groupings "represent two different ways of describing the same clinical entity **(p. 293)**."

16.28 The answer is **E**. Lipowski identified four factors predisposing people to hypochondriasis: genetics, developmental learning, personality, and sociocultural environment **(p. 294)**.

16.29 The answer is **B**. Theories of hypochondriasis as a learned behavior suggest that children learn that suffering from a "physical" illness

Somatoform and Psychosexual Disorders **101**

results in anxious attention from parents and allows them to avoid unpleasant duties **(p. 294)**.

16.30 The answer is **E**. Studies of elderly hypochondriacal patients identified the following factors as contributing to the development of the disorders: recurrent exposure to criticism in a situation that provides no possibility of escape, reduction in economic status, loss of spouse and friends, isolation due to socioeconomic factors, and deterioration in marital satisfaction **(p. 294)**.

16.31 The answer is **B**. Treatment techniques for the hypochondriacal patient must recognize that the hypochondriacal symptoms are an unconscious defense mechanism providing a pattern of social adjustment and maintenance of self-esteem. The therapist should not give a false diagnosis because the patient's symptoms will persist and the doctor-patient relationship will be damaged. Supportive statements are helpful in conveying the physician's concern and willingness to work with the patient to relieve the patient's symptoms, such as the following: 1) "The results of this workup indicate that there is no adequate explanation for your symptoms. It is obvious that you are having problems and I will be pleased to work with you to improve your situation." 2) "I'm sure it would be reassuring if I had a specific diagnosis, but I don't. However, I am willing to follow your case carefully and will try to find some way to improve your health and well-being." Such statements include supportive remarks and avoid threats to the hypochondriacal defense. Only 2.4% of physicians treating hypochondriacal patients use placebo medication. Such agents have been found to be useful in practice and research **(pp. 296–297)**.

16.32 The answer is **A**. The elderly hypochondriacal patient may believe that the psychiatrist's role is to determine or demonstrate that his or her physical symptoms are of mental origin. These patients confront the psychiatrist by asserting that nervousness or imagination play no role in their symptoms. Hostility toward a prior physician may be expressed as well. The treating psychiatrist should 1) state that he or she recognizes that other individuals may have indicated that the symptoms were of mental or emotional cause and that this is understandably upsetting to the patient, as well as emphasize the role of the psychiatrist as being involved with the total health and well-being of the individual; 2) not defend the prior physician but confine his or her remarks to a recognition that the patient's experiences have been both upsetting and disappointing **(p. 298)**.

16.33 The answer is **B**. Among older patients age 70 and over who suffered a myocardial infarction, 30% did not experience pain as a major presenting complaint. Elderly patients with appendicitis experience generalized abdominal pain localized to the right lower quadrant associated with nausea and vomiting, but fever and leukocytosis may be lacking. Persistent pain in the elderly is associated with physical disorders seen frequently in late life, including osteoarthritis, rheumatic arthritis, angina of effort, herpes zoster, and gout **(p. 300)**.

16.34 The answer is **E**. Although chronic pain cannot be eliminated in the elderly, the intensity and frequency of pain exacerbations can be decreased. Functional capacity can be restored, and mood and quality of life can be improved **(p. 302)**.

16.35 The answer is **A**. Testosterone replacement must be done with caution. Testosterone frequently exacerbates BPH and is contraindicated if carcinoma of the prostate is suspected. The hormone can accelerate the development of carcinoma. Because testosterone can produce polycythemia, regular hemoglobin and red cell determination must be monitored frequently **(pp. 303–304)**.

16.36 The answer is **A**. Sexual activity continues in late life and is maintained until after age 75 between marital partners. Although earlier studies (1950s) found that better socioeconomic status was associated with continuation of sexual activity, this may have been related to better socioeconomic status being associated with better health. Factors identified as affecting the continuation of sexual activity included the availability of a sexual partner, the physical and mental health of the partners, and the pattern of sexual interest and activity established in early adulthood **(p. 304)**.

16.37 The answer is **C**. Painful intercourse in older women is usually due to estrogen deficiency. A sexually inactive woman in her 70s should resume intercourse with preparation that may include mechanical dilation as well as hormonal replacement therapy in order to return to sexual functioning without discomfort or injury. A diseased, retroverted uterus may be a source of pain as well **(p. 306)**.

16.38 The answer is **E**. Sexual behavioral problems among elderly nursing home residents include exposure of genitalia and masturbation. Among institutionalized elderly persons, the elders' interest and attitude toward sexuality are based on their prior interest and attitude as well as their prior level of sexual activity. Sexual behavior between nursing home residents can mobilize "paternalistic tendencies in staff."

When a nondemented or mildly demented resident pursues another nursing home resident who is more demented, the nursing home staff may view these residents as the perpetrator and the victim. Resolution of such staff/resident conflicts requires staff meetings where staff members can express their discomfort and be helped to understand that a resident's activity is not to be limited by someone else's moral values **(p. 308)**.

Chapter 17

Bereavement and Adjustment Disorders

QUESTIONS

Directions: **Select the single best response for each of the following questions.**

17.1 *Bereavement* is best defined as

    A. The normal losses occurring in late life.
    B. The reaction that results after the death of someone close.
    C. An adjustment disorder with depressed features.
    D. All of these.
    E. None of these.

17.2 Various authors have suggested different responses to the process of handling loss

    A. Surrendering psychological attachment to the lost object.
    B. Attempting to unite with the lost object.
    C. Completing a series of stages or phases of adaptation to the lost object resulting in reinvestment of the psychic energy into another person or activity.
    D. All of these.
    E. None of these.

17.3 The course of grieving proceeds

    A. In an orderly fashion from one phase to another phase in the adaptation to loss.
    B. Varies from person to person.
    C. Can become a complex process.
    D. All of these.
    E. None of these.

17.4 Symptoms seen in normal grieving are
- A. Guilt over things done or not done at the time of death of the loved one.
- B. Thoughts that the person should have died when the loved one died.
- C. Thoughts that the survivor would be better off dead.
- D. All of these.
- E. None of these.

17.5 Substantial recovery from an episode of bereavement should occur within
- A. 2 weeks.
- B. 2 months.
- C. 2 years.
- D. All of these.
- E. None of these.

17.6 The experience of grief, the psychological distress, and the level of grief remain high for
- A. 30 months after the death.
- B. 15 months after the death.
- C. 6 months after the death.
- D. All of these.
- E. None of these.

17.7 Risk factors that intensify the grief experience include
- A. Age and gender.
- B. Social isolation.
- C. Violent or unexpected death.
- D. All of these.
- E. None of these.

17.8 When the grieving process is complicated by the presence of a major depressive disorder, it is important to
- A. Allow the grieving process to continue.
- B. Initiate treatment of the major depressive disorder.
- C. Wait 6 months to see if the depression resolves.
- D. All of these.
- E. None of these.

Bereavement and Adjustment Disorders

17.9 The tasks of grief counseling include
 A. Accepting the reality of the loss.
 B. Experiencing the pain of grief.
 C. Adjusting to an environment in which the loved one is no longer there.
 D. All of these.
 E. None of these.

17.10 The DSM-IV criteria for a diagnosis of an adjustment disorder require
 A. Clinically significant emotional or behavioral symptoms.
 B. An identifiable psychosocial stressor.
 C. Onset of symptoms within 3 months after the stressor.
 D. All of these.
 E. None of these.

17.11 An adjustment disorder is defined as *chronic* if it
 A. Persists for 6 months or less.
 B. Persists for more than 6 months.
 C. Resolves within 6 months after the termination of the stressor.
 D. All of these.
 E. None of these.

Directions: **For each of the statements below, one or more of the answers is correct. Choose**

 A. If 1, 2, and 3 are correct.
 B. If only 1 and 3 are correct.
 C. If only 2 and 4 are correct.
 D. If only 4 is correct.
 E. If all are correct.

17.12 In models that describe phases or stages of grief, specific symptoms associated with the second phase of grieving include
 1. Frequent crying and chronic sleep disturbance.
 2. Blue mood and poor appetite.
 3. Low energy and feelings of fatigue.
 4. Problems with attention and concentration.

17.13 The primary factor of importance in an adjustment disorder is
1. The type of stressor(s).
2. The number of losses.
3. The presence of a social network.
4. The way the individual copes.

17.14 Forms of coping used by the elderly include
1. Intrapersonal, emotion-focused coping.
2. Active, interpersonal coping.
3. Distancing, acceptance of responsibility, and positive reappraisal.
4. Escapist fantasy.

ANSWERS

17.1 The answer is **B.** *Bereavement* is the term used to describe the reaction or process that results after the death of someone close **(pp. 313–314)**.

17.2 The answer is **D.** Several authors have developed various theoretical perspectives to explain how people respond to significant loss. Freud (1917/1957), in *Mourning and Melancholia,* identified the primary task of mourning as the gradual surrender of psychological attachment to the deceased. In his attachment theory, Bowlby (1961) emphasized that bereavement results in many types of attachment behavior that function to reunite the person with the lost object. Parkes (1972) and Horowitz (1976) proposed models of grieving composed of phases or stages of adaptation to the lost object **(p. 314)**, with the final phase of adaptation to the loss resulting in the disengagement of some or most of the psychic energy and reinvestment of that energy in other persons and activities **(p. 315)**.

17.3 The answer is **B.** The course of grieving differs in people. The manifestation of grief they experience and the order and speed with which they move through the grieving process differ from individual to individual **(p. 315)**.

17.4 The answer is **E.** None of these symptoms is seen in a "normal" grief reaction. Symptoms identified by DSM-IV as being inconsistent with a "normal" grief reaction include guilt over things done or not done at the time of death of the loved one, thoughts that the person should have

Bereavement and Adjustment Disorders 109

died when the loved one died, and thoughts that the survivor would be better off dead **(p. 316)**.

17.5 The answer is **C**. Substantial recovery from an episode of bereavement should occur within the "typical" span of 2 years **(p. 317)**.

17.6 The answer is **A**. The experience of grief, the psychological distress, and the level of grief remained high over the length of a 30-month interval after the spouse's death **(p. 318)**.

17.7 The answer is **B**. Risk factors (variables) that were found to intensify the grief experience included age (older persons adapted better to loss), gender (men were at higher risk), mode of death, presence of significant depression shortly after the death, self-esteem and perceived coping, prior relationship satisfaction, and social support (socially isolated males were more at risk) **(pp. 319–320)**.

17.8 The answer is **B**. When another significant psychiatric disorder (depression, substance abuse, generalized anxiety disorder) is complicating the grieving process, that disorder should be treated first with medication and/or psychotherapy **(p. 321)**.

17.9 The answer is **D**. The tasks of grief counseling include helping the bereaved person with accepting the reality of the loss, experiencing the pain of grief, adjusting to an environment in which the loved one is truly no longer there, and emotionally detaching sufficiently from the decreased to be able to resume a normal life **(p. 322)**.

17.10 The answer is **D**. DSM-IV defines an *adjustment disorder* as "clinically significant emotional or behavioral symptoms in response to an identifiable psychosocial stressor(s) that develops within 3 months after the onset of the stressor(s)" **(p. 323)**.

17.11 The answer is **B**. By definition based on DSM-IV criteria, an adjustment disorder is chronic if it persists for more than 6 months **(p. 323)**.

17.12 The answer is **A**. Symptoms associated with the second phase of grieving include frequent crying, chronic sleep disturbance, blue mood, poor appetite, low energy, feelings of fatigue, loss of interest in daily living, and problems with attention and concentration. Despite the fact that certain symptoms of grief and depression overlap, most grieving elders do not develop a major depressive disorder **(p. 314)**.

17.13 The answer is **D**. How an individual copes with the stress of losses rather than the losses themselves is of primary importance **(p. 324)**.

17.14 The answer is **B**. The elderly use intrapersonal, emotion-focused forms of coping involving distancing, acceptance of responsibility, and positive reappraisal. In contrast, younger persons use more active, interpersonal, problem-focused forms of coping. Older persons were found to be less hostile in reaction to negative events and less likely to rely on escapist fantasy **(p. 325)**.

CHAPTER 18

Sleep and Chronobiological Disturbances

QUESTIONS

Directions: **Select the single best response for each of the following questions.**

18.1 Factors affecting healthy sleep in the elderly include

   A. Comorbid medical and neuropsychiatric disorders.
   B. Psychosocial factors (retirement and bereavement).
   C. Normal age-related changes in sleep and circadian physiology.
   D. All of these.
   E. None of these.

18.2 Insomnia has been found to be associated with

   A. Alcoholism.
   B. Anxiety disorders.
   C. Depression.
   D. All of these.
   E. None of these.

18.3 Rapid eye movement (REM) sleep is composed of

   A. Stages 1, 2, and 3.
   B. Stages 3 and 4 only.
   C. Stages 1 and 2 only.
   D. All of these.
   E. None of these.

18.4 Specific changes in sleep that occur between the third and ninth decades of life include
   A. Reduction in electroencephalogram (EEG) amplitude.
   B. Increase in the number of microarousals and awakenings.
   C. Reduction and disappearance of visually scored slow-wave sleep.
   D. All of these.
   E. None of these.

18.5 Older patients
   A. Have decreased nocturnal sleep.
   B. Take more naps.
   C. Have sleep-disordered breathing and nocturnal myoclonus.
   D. All of these.
   E. None of these.

18.6 Among the elderly, the circadian oscillator
   A. Is phase advanced by 90 minutes.
   B. Is phase retarded by 60 minutes.
   C. Is phase null.
   D. All of these.
   E. None of these.

18.7 The acquisition of the behavior of napping during the day by older persons is due to
   A. Retirement.
   B. The absence of a structured daytime schedule.
   C. Complaints of nocturnal insomnia.
   D. All of these.
   E. None of these.

18.8 Sleep-disordered breathing or obstructive sleep apnea is a collapse of the oropharynx during respiration resulting in hypoxia and sleep fragmentation. Symptoms include
   A. Hypersomnia.
   B. Decreased alertness.
   C. Decreased concentration and attention.
   D. All of these.
   E. None of these.

18.9 A sleep parameter predictive of mortality in the elderly is
   A. The number of obstructive events per hour of sleep.
   B. The total sleep time in a 24-hour period.
   C. The number of REM cycles in a 24-hour period.
   D. All of these.
   E. None of these.

18.10 The prevalence of periodic leg movements ranges from
   A. 25%–75%.
   B. 37.5 %–57%.
   C. 20%–40%.
   D. All of these.
   E. None of these.

18.11 One explanation for the sleep disturbance observed in patients with Alzheimer's disease is
   A. Degeneration of the brain stem region and associated pathways involved in the sleep-wake cycle.
   B. Increase in hippocampal cortical neurons.
   C. Increase in presynaptic cholinergic neurons.
   D. All of these.
   E. None of these.

18.12 "Sundowning," a transient nocturnal delirium, is characterized by
   A. Restlessness and agitation.
   B. Decreased ability to maintain attention.
   C. Hallucinations and illusions.
   D. All of these.
   E. None of these.

18.13 Behavioral treatment of "sundowning" includes
   A. Reorientation.
   B. Reassurance.
   C. Use of a night light.
   D. All of these.
   E. None of these.

18.14 Of patients with Parkinson's disease,
- A. 25% have a sleep problem.
- B. 55% have a sleep problem.
- C. 75% have a sleep problem.
- D. All of these.
- E. None of these.

18.15 A high dose of L-dopa/carbidopa at bedtime can
- A. Increase sleep latency.
- B. Disrupt sleep in the first half of the night.
- C. Promote sleep in the second half of the night.
- D. All of these.
- E. None of these.

Directions: **For each of the statements below, one or more of the answers is correct. Choose**

- A. If 1, 2, and 3 are correct.
- B. If only 1 and 3 are correct.
- C. If only 2 and 4 are correct.
- D. If only 4 is correct.
- E. If all are correct.

18.16 Sleep is divided into
1. REM sleep.
2. Stages 3 and 4.
3. Non-REM sleep.
4. Sleep latency.

18.17 During REM sleep, the following are observed:
1. Increased brain electrical activity.
2. Increased cerebral blood flow above the awake state.
3. Fluctuations of eye movement and heart rate.
4. Generalized muscle atonia.

18.18 Slow-wave sleep is defined by
1. Frequency.
2. Pitch.
3. Amplitude.
4. Volume.

Sleep and Chronobiological Disturbances 115

18.19 A higher mortality rate is seen in persons who
1. Are depressed.
2. Are cognitively impaired.
3. Have reduced REM sleep.
4. Have a decreased percentage of substance abuse

18.20 Gender differences found in sleep studies reported that
1. Elderly men had more awakenings and less slow-wave sleep.
2. Elderly women had more sleep awakenings and less slow-wave sleep.
3. Elderly men had the onset of slow-wave sleep reduction sooner than elderly women.
4. Elderly women had the onset of slow-wave sleep reduction sooner than older men.

18.21 The prevalence of sleep disordered breathing is
1. 50% of community-dwelling elderly.
2. 24% of community-dwelling elderly.
3. 72% of institutionalized elderly.
4. 42% of institutionalized elderly.

18.22 Depressed older patients were found to have
1. Decreased slow-wave sleep.
2. Reduced REM latency.
3. Increased phasic REM activity in the first half of the night.
4. Prominent sleep continuity disturbance.

18.23 Older persons with probable Alzheimer's disease were found to have
1. A disturbed sleep-wake cycle.
2. Night time wandering.
3. Insomnia.
4. Nighttime delirium ("sundowning").

18.24 Nonpharmacologic treatment of sleep disorders involves education of the patient about sleep hygiene that includes
1. Adhering to a regular sleep-wake schedule.
2. Avoiding stimulants and alcohol.
3. Limiting daytime naps.
4. Getting regular exercise.

18.25 Two techniques involved in promoting healthy sleep include
1. Stimulus control behavior modification.
2. Psychosocial modification.
3. Sleep restriction therapy.
4. Total sleep therapy.

18.26 Benzodiapines with an intermediate half-life without active metabolites are widely used in the treatment of insomnia. These include
1. Lorazepam.
2. Oxazepam.
3. Temezapam.
4. Diazepam.

18.27 Antidepressants used to treat insomnia include
1. Nortriptyline.
2. Trazodone.
3. Desipramine.
4. Zolpidem.

ANSWERS

18.1 The answer is **D**. Assessment of sleep disorders in the elderly must recognize the factors that affect healthy sleep in the elderly. These factors include comorbid medical and neuropsychiatric disorders, psychosocial factors (retirement, isolation), and normal age-related changes in sleep and circadian physiology **(p. 329)**.

18.2 The answer is **C**. Several longitudinal studies have documented an association between complaints of insomnia and depressed mood. Data from the Epidemiologic Catchment Area survey found sleep complaints often preceded the onset of mood disorder. Thus, early evaluation and early intervention for insomnia may prevent subsequent depression **(p. 330)**.

18.3 The answer is **E**. REM sleep is rapid eye movement sleep. Non-REM sleep is divided into Stages 1, 2, 3, and 4, with stages 3 and 4 defined as *slow-wave* or *delta sleep* **(p. 330)**.

18.4 The answer is **E**. Older persons tend to sleep only 70%–80% of the time that they are in bed. Primary changes occurring between the third and

Sleep and Chronobiological Disturbances 117

ninth decade of life include a reduction in EEG amplitude, a reduction and disappearance of visually scored slow-wave sleep, and an increase in the number of microarousals and awakenings **(p. 330)**.

18.5 The answer is **D**. Studies of sleep in the elderly have suggested that the segregation of sleep and wakefulness in the light-dark cycle breaks down with age, but the higher prevalence of sleep-disordered breathing and nocturnal myoclonus seen in the elderly may contribute to these findings. Older people do have decreased nocturnal sleep and take naps during the day. Some 80% of the elderly nap during the day **(p. 330)**.

18.6 The answer is **A**. Temperature, REM sleep, and cortisol rhythm, all thought to reflect the underlying circadian oscillator, are phase advanced by approximately 90 minutes in the elderly compared with younger control subjects **(p. 331)**.

18.7 The answer is **D**. Retirement results frequently in the loss of a structured daytime schedule. Napping during the day can become a new behavior that results in less sleep at night resulting in complaints of nocturnal insomnia **(p. 331)**.

18.8 The answer is **D**. Symptoms of obstructive sleep apnea include hypersomnolence, decreased alertness, diminished concentration and attention, systemic and pulmonary hypertension, and cor pulmonale **(p. 332)**.

18.9 The answer is **A**. The number of obstructive events per hour of sleep was found to predict mortality in the elderly **(p. 332)**.

18.10 The answer is **B**. Estimates of the prevalence of periodic leg movements in healthy elderly people range from 37.5% to 57% **(p. 332)**.

18.11 The answer is **A**. The sleep disturbance observed in patients with dementia has been explained as due to a degeneration of the brain stem region and associated pathways involved in the sleep-wake cycle. Alzheimer's disease results in a decrease in hippocampal and cortical neurons as well as a decrease in presynaptic cholinergic neurons **(p. 333)**.

18.12 The answer is **D**. "Sundowning" may be best conceptualized as a transient nocturnal delirium that is characterized by decreased ability to maintain attention, disorientation, disorganized thoughts and speech, restlessness and agitation, hallucinations and illusions, anxiety, paranoia, and mood lability **(p. 333)**.

18.13 The answer is **D**. Reorientation, reassurance, and the use of a low-level night light can be helpful to older demented patients with transient nocturnal delirium. If mediation is used, low-dose, high-potency antipsychotic medications are often helpful **(p. 333)**.

18.14 The answer is **C**. Some 75% of patients with Parkinson's disease will experience sleep problems. They have difficulty initiating sleep, experience nocturnal vocalizations, apneic episodes, spontaneous daytime napping, difficulty turning over in bed, and sometimes REM sleep behavior disorder **(p. 334)**.

18.15 The answer is **D**. High-dose L-dopa/carbidopa at bedtime affects sleep architecture. Sleep latency is increased, sleep in the first half of the night is disrupted, and sleep in the second half of the night is promoted. Dopaminergic medication may cause vivid dreams, nightmares, or night terror **(p. 334)**.

18.16 The answer is **B**. Normal sleep is divided into REM and non-REM sleep **(p. 330)**.

18.17 The answer is **E**. During REM sleep, there is relatively increased brain electrical activity. Increased cerebral blood flow above the awake state is found as well as fluctuations of eye movements, heart rate, and respirations. A generalized muscle atonia is observed in which the subject is paralyzed except for the diaphragm and the extraocular muscles **(p. 330)**.

18.18 The answer is **B**. *Slow-wave sleep* is defined by both frequency and amplitude parameters. With increasing age, a substantial reduction occurs in the EEG amplitude resulting in the reduction or loss of visually scored slow-wave sleep **(p. 330)**.

18.19 The answer is **A**. A higher mortality rate was found in depressed, cognitively impaired elderly patients with reduced REM sleep. Elderly persons in general have an increased percentage of Stage 1 sleep because of the increased number of microarousals that they experience **(p. 330)**.

18.20 The answer is **B**. Although elderly women used more sedative hypnotic medications and had more subjective complaints of insomnia, older men were found to have more awakenings and less slow-wave sleep than older women. Older men also had the onset of slow-wave sleep reductions sooner than older women **(p. 331)**.

Sleep and Chronobiological Disturbances **119**

18.21 The answer is **C**. Approximately 24% of community-dwelling elderly and 42% of institutionalized elderly persons have sleep-disordered breathing **(p. 332)**.

18.22 The answer is **E**. The sleep disturbance found in depressed patients included decreased slow-wave sleep, reduced REM latency, increased phasic REM activity in the first half of the night, and prominent sleep continuity disturbance **(p. 332)**.

18.23 The answer is **E**. Patients with probable Alzheimer's disease exhibit a disturbed sleep-wake cycle, nighttime wandering, insomnia, and nighttime delirium ("Sundowning"), which often results in institutionalization **(p. 333)**.

18.24 The answer is **E**. Sleep hygiene, part of the education of the patient in good sleep habits, emphasizes adhering to a regular sleep-wake cycle, avoiding stimulants and alcohol, and limiting daytime naps **(p. 335)**.

18.25 The answer is **B**. Two strategies promoting healthy sleep involve reducing the time spent awake in bed. These two strategies are the stimulus control behavior modification approach (going to bed only when sleepy, limiting the use of the bed for sleep and intimacy, getting out of bed if not asleep in 15 minutes) and the sleep restriction therapy approach (limiting the time in bed to the estimated sleep time) **(p. 335)**.

18.26 The answer is **A**. Lorazepam, oxazepam, and temazepam are benzodiazepines with an intermediate half-life and without an active metabolite. They usually produce little daytime sedation and are eliminated in the elderly in 8–15 hours **(p. 335)**. Unlike diazepam, whose active metabolite (desmethyldiazepam) has a half-life of 90–110 hours, the intermediate benzodiazepines are less likely to accumulate and will not produce the excessive sedation and cognitive or motor impairment caused by benzodiazepines with longer half-lives such as diazepam **(pp. 335–336)**.

18.27 The answer is **A**. Secondary tricyclic amines (nortriptyline and desipramine) are less anticholinergic and less likely to produce orthostatic hypotension. Trazodone, a heterocyclic antidepressant, has few anticholinergic properties but has significant alpha-adrenergic properties. It is quite sedating and is associated with hypotension. Zolpidem is a newer nonbenzodiazepine imidazopyridine-class hypnotic agent that has been found to be effective in inducing and maintaining sleep. It is rapidly absorbed in just over 2 hours and has a half-life of 2.9 hours in the elderly. It has not been associated with daytime sleepiness or memory effects. It is highly bound to plasma protein and does not accumulate. It has no muscle relaxant, anxiolytic, or anticonvulsant effects **(p. 336)**.

CHAPTER 19

Alcohol and Drug Problems

QUESTIONS

Directions: **Select the single best response for each of the following questions.**

19.1 The prevalence of alcohol use/dependence for men age 65 and older ranges from
   A. 1% to 3%.
   B. 2% to 5%.
   C. 3% to 7%.
   D. All of these.
   E. None of these.

19.2 The prevalence of alcohol abuse/dependence among women age 65 and older ranges from
   A. 0.1% to 0.7%.
   B. 0.3% to 1.1%.
   C. 0.5% to 1.5%.
   D. All of these.
   E. None of these.

19.3 Risk factors for alcohol abuse in the elderly are
   A. Male gender and poor education.
   B. Low income.
   C. A history of depression.
   D. All of these.
   E. None of these.

19.4 The comorbidity of alcohol problems and psychiatric illness in late life is
   A. 5%–10%.
   B. 10%–15%.
   C. 15%–20%.
   D. All of these.
   E. None of these.

19.5 The current cohort of older persons was raised in a culture with a strong tradition of temperance. Abstinence is reported to be
   A. 52% in men and 68% in women.
   B. 42% in men and 58% in women.
   C. 32% in men and 48% in women.
   D. All of these.
   E. None of these.

19.6 Characteristics of older alcoholics include
   A. Poorer health.
   B. More physical problems.
   C. More problems with finances and social isolation.
   D. All of these.
   E. None of these.

19.7 Older adults have
   A. More total body water.
   B. More extracellular fluid.
   C. Lower total body fat.
   D. All of these.
   E. None of these.

19.8 The hepatic enzyme that oxidizes alcohol is
   A. Alcohol dehydrogenase.
   B. Alcohol acetaldehyde.
   C. Adenosine diphosphate.
   D. All of these.
   E. None of these.

19.9 The reduction of nicotinamide adenine dinucleotide (NAD)
   A. Enhances lipid synthesis in the liver.
   B. Increases esterification of fatty acids.
   C. Decreases protein accumulation.
   D. All of these.
   E. None of these.

19.10 Among persons age 65 and older, the eighth leading cause of death is
   A. Stroke.
   B. Accidents.
   C. Cirrhosis.
   D. All of these.
   E. None of these.

19.11 Peripheral neuropathy due to the deficiency of thiamine and other B-complex vitamins may occur in
   A. 45% of chronic alcoholic patients.
   B. 35% of chronic alcoholic patients.
   C. 25% of chronic alcoholic patients.
   D. All of these.
   E. None of these.

19.12 The relatively rapid metabolism of alcohol compared with most sedative hypnotics may produce
   A. Rebound awakening 3–4 hours into sleep.
   B. Difficulty in falling asleep.
   C. Visual hallucinations.
   D. All of these.
   E. None of these.

19.13 The tremulous state of the alcohol withdrawal syndrome peaks within
   A. 1–2 days.
   B. 3–4 days.
   C. 5–6 days.
   D. All of these.
   E. None of these.

19.14 Diagnostic evaluations of the older adult with a suspected alcohol problem should include
   A. A detailed history from the patient and family members.
   B. A physical examination assessing liver size and the presence of peripheral neuropathy.
   C. A thorough review of psychiatric symptoms, particularly cognitive status.
   D. All of these.
   E. None of these.

19.15 Data for persons age 65 and older from the Epidemiologic Catchment Area survey found in
   A. Two of three sites: no evidence of abuse.
   B. One of three sites: a prevalence of abuse of 0.2%.
   C. Three of three sites: a lifetime prevalence of abuse of 0.1%
   D. All of these.
   E. None of these.

Directions: **For each of the statements below, one or more of the answers is correct. Choose**

   A. If 1, 2, and 3 are correct.
   B. If only 1 and 3 are correct.
   C. If only 2 and 4 are correct.
   D. If only 4 is correct.
   E. If all are correct.

19.16 In the metabolism of alcohol,
   1. Peak blood levels are reached within 30–90 minutes after alcohol intake.
   2. Complete absorption can take from 2 to 6 hours.
   3. Most food in the stomach, especially milk and milk products, retard the absorption of alcohol.
   4. Alcohol absorption in the elderly is slower than at earlier stages of the life cycle.

19.17 Persons with chronic alcoholism have
   1. Lower basal gastric acid output and a maximal acid output.
   2. A decline in absorption of folic acid and vitamin B_{12}.
   3. Protein malnutrition.
   4. Iron deficiency.

19.18 End-stage alcoholic dementia is characterized by
   1. Relatively intact intellectual functioning.
   2. Severe anterograde amnesia.
   3. Severe retrograde amnesia.
   4. Incontinence.

Alcohol and Drug Problems

19.19 *Addiction* is defined as a behavioral pattern of drug use characterized by
   1. Overwhelming involvement with the use of a drug.
   2. Securing a supply of the drug.
   3. A high tendency to relapse after withdrawal.
   4. Suicide attempts.

19.20 Treatment of the older persons with alcohol abuse/dependence should include
   1. Restoration of fluid and electrolyte imbalance.
   2. Assessment for magnesium deficiency.
   3. Use of diazepam to manage alcohol withdrawal.
   4. Involvement of the patient's family.

19.21 The acetaldehyde syndrome involves
   1. Facial flushing and nausea and vomiting.
   2. Intense throbbing in the head and neck.
   3. Difficulty breathing and blurred vision.
   4. Hypertension and chest pain.

19.22 Self-help groups, such as Alcoholic Anonymous (AA), may be rejected by the older person because of a self-sufficient attitude. An alternative to AA involves
   1. Mobilizing social network resources (church, membership in community groups).
   2. Coordinating health care services (visiting nurse, physicians and therapists).
   3. Using behavioral therapy.
   4. Participating in educational programs.

19.23 Factors contributing to prescription drug abuse/dependence in the current cohort of elderly persons include
   1. Hesitancy to ask questions resulting in confusion about how to take the prescribed medications.
   2. Use of borrowed medications to cut costs.
   3. Use of over-the-counter medications.
   4. Physicians' response to "do something" or to prescribe "defensively."

ANSWERS

19.1 The answer is **B**. The prevalence of alcohol abuse/dependence among men age 65 and older ranges from 1.9% (2%) to 4.6% (5%) **(p. 342)**.

19.2 The answer is **A**. The prevalence of alcohol abuse/dependence among women age 65 and older ranges from 0.1 to 0.7% **(p. 342)**.

19.3 The answer is **D**. In the elderly and for the general population risk factors for alcohol abuse are similar: male gender, poor education, low income, and a history of other psychiatric disorders, especially depression **(p. 342)**.

19.4 The answer is **B**. The comorbidity of alcohol problems and psychiatric illness in late life is 10%–15% **(p. 342)**.

19.5 The answer is **A**. Some 52% of elderly men and 68% of elderly women reported that they were abstainers from the use of alcohol in a cohort of older persons who were raised in a culture with a strong tradition of temperance **(p. 342)**.

19.6 The answer is **D**. Characteristics of older alcoholics identified by Rathbone-McCuan et al. (1976) included poorer health, more physical problems, more problems with finances, and social isolation **(p. 343)**.

19.7 The answer is **E**. Age-related physiologic changes observed in older persons include a decrease in total body water, less extracellular fluid, and a higher percentage of total body fat. Thus, a standard ingested dose of alcohol will result in a higher blood level in an older adult than in a younger adult because of the lower effective fluid volume for distribution **(p. 343)**.

19.8 The answer is **A**. The hepatic enzyme that oxidizes alcohol is alcohol dehydrogenase. Age does not effect the function of this enzyme, which is slow and constant in its action **(pp. 343–344)**.

19.9 The answer is **A**. The reduction of NAD to NADH enhances lipid synthesis in the liver. The oxidation of alcohol in the liver produces a relative increase in NADH. The increase in acetylglycerophosphate stimulates the esterification of fatty acids, which leads to a collection of fat in the liver. The accumulation of fat and an accompanying accumulation of protein eventually cannot be reversed and progresses to various stages of liver disease, especially cirrhosis **(p. 344)**.

Alcohol and Drug Problems **127**

19.10 The answer is **C**. Among persons age 65 and older, the eighth leading cause of death is cirrhosis **(p. 344)**. Undernutrition resulting from chronic alcohol intake commonly leads to cirrhosis in a person who uses large amounts of alcohol over long periods of time (the "skid row alcoholic") **(p. 344)**.

19.11 The answer is **A**. Peripheral neuropathy due to the deficiency of thiamine and other B-complex vitamins may occur in 45% of chronic alcoholic patients **(p. 345)**.

19.12 The answer is **A**. The relatively rapid metabolism of alcohol compared with most sedative hypnotics may produce rebound awakening at a point 3–4 hours into sleep. The older adult who uses alcohol falls asleep without difficulty but experiences disruption of his or her sleep during the night **(p. 346)**. Visual hallucinations are seen in alcohol withdrawal **(p. 349)**.

19.13 The answer is **A**. The tremulous state of the alcohol withdrawal syndrome peaks within 1–2 days **(p. 347)**.

19.14 The answer is **D**. The diagnostic evaluation of the older adult suspected of alcohol problems should include a detailed history from the patient and family. The physical examination should assess hepatic size and neurologic function, particularly episodes of amnesia and the presence of peripheral neuropathies. A thorough review of psychiatric symptoms, particularly cognitive function, should be completed **(pp. 347–348)**.

19.15 The answer is **D**. Data from three of the five sites of the Epidemiologic Catchment Area survey found no drug abuse in two of three sites and a prevalence of 0.2% in the third site. The lifetime prevalence of drug abuse/dependence across the three sites was 0.1% **(p. 352)**.

19.16 The answer is **A**. Peak blood levels of ethyl alcohol are reached within 30–90 minutes after alcohol intake. Complete absorption may take from 2 to 6 hours. Alcohol absorption is rapid in the elderly as it is in younger ages. In the stomach, most foods, particularly milk and milk products, retard the absorption of alcohol **(p. 343)**.

19.17 The answer is **E**. Persons with chronic alcoholism have a lower basal gastric acid output and a maximal acid output that increases the likelihood of developing chronic atrophic gastritis. The atrophic gastritis may facilitate the formation of gastric mucosal lesions, which lead to upper gastrointestinal bleeding. Chronic alcohol use produces a decline in the absorption of both folic acid and vitamin B_{12}. These deficiencies can produce cognitive and psychological manifestations in chronic alcoholics with muscle wasting, hypoproteinemia, and edema **(p. 345)**.

19.18 The answer is **A**. End-stage alcoholic dementia is characterized by relatively intact intellectual functioning and severe antegrade and retrograde amnesia **(p. 345)**.

19.19 The answer is **A**. *Addiction* is defined by Jaffe (1980) as "a behavioral pattern of drug use, characterized by overwhelming involvement with the use of a drug (compulsive use), the securing of its supply, and a high tendency to relapse after withdrawal" **(p. 346)**.

19.20 The answer is **E**. The treatment of the older person with alcohol abuse/dependence should include the involvement of the patient's family during detoxification and for the long-term goal of abstinence. In the severely alcoholic elder, restoration of fluid and electrolyte balance is essential. The use of glucose solutions should be avoided because they can result in iatrogenic increase in glucose to diabetic levels because of the high carbohydrate diet of the alcohol-dependent elder. Because chronic alcoholics suffer from magnesium deficiency, magnesium levels should be assessed and replaced if indicated. A medication that is cross-tolerant with alcohol should be used (e.g., diazepam) to prevent withdrawal **(p. 349)**.

19.21 The answer is **E**. Disulfiram can be an important agent in preventing relapse in alcohol-dependent persons. It should be administered daily by a family member. Its use requires a contract between the patient, the physician, and at least one family member. The acetaldehyde syndrome results from an increase in acetaldehyde when ethanol and disulfiram are present concurrently. Symptoms include flushing of the face, intense throbbing headache, difficulty in breathing, nausea, vomiting, sweating, thirst, chest pain, hypertension, vertigo, blurred vision, and confusion **(p. 350)**.

19.22 The answer is **E**. Because of the self-sufficient attitude of the current cohort of older persons, participation in self-help groups such as AA may be rejected. An alternative to AA involves incorporating the required components of treatment in an integrated approach by the utilization of social network resources (church, membership in community groups), health services (visiting nurses, coordination between physicians and therapists), the use of behavioral therapy, and participation in educational programs **(p. 350)**.

19.23 The answer is **E**. Factors contributing to prescription drug abuse/dependence in the elderly include the hesitancy of the older person to ask questions resulting in confusion about how to take medication. The passive older person may use drugs prescribed by several physicians and not question even the prescription of the same drug by two different physicians. Due to limited finances, an older person may borrow medications from a friend with similar complaints. The use of over-the-counter medications may produce drug-drug interactions (e.g., diphenhydramine with tricyclic antidepressants) that can produce anticholinergic toxicity. Patients expect physicians to "do something" for a consultation—usually a prescription. Physicians covering nursing homes or long-term care facilities are called by nursing staff and family members about behavioral symptoms (agitation and sleep problems). The physician's "defensive" prescribing is the result of managing an acutely agitated and cognitively impaired older adult in a facility with limited personnel **(pp. 352–353)**.

SECTION IV

Treatment of Psychiatric Disorders in Late Life

CHAPTER 20

Pharmacological Treatment

QUESTIONS

Directions: **Select the single best response for each of the following questions.**

20.1 Elderly individuals frequently take multiple medications, which leads to
   A. Compliance problems.
   B. Drug-drug interactions.
   C. Iatrogenic illness.
   D. All of these.
   E. None of these.

20.2 The age-related decline in renal function and perfusion affects the metabolism of medications that are excreted by the kidney. Specific medications affected include
   A. Lithium.
   B. Dextroamphetamine.
   C. Fluvoxamine.
   D. All of these.
   E. None of these.

20.3 The presentation of early-onset schizophrenia changes with age, and the older patient exhibits
   A. Withdrawal.
   B. Agitation.
   C. Bizarre hallucinations.
   D. All of these.
   E. None of these.

20.4 Aliphatic phenothiazines
   A. Are specific in their effect.
   B. Are low potency.
   C. Affect only the dopamine pathway.
   D. All of these.
   E. None of these.

20.5 Piperidine phenothiazines are preferred in the elderly because of their
   A. Sedating properties.
   B. Methylation of their tertiary amines.
   C. Anticholinergic properties.
   D. All of these.
   E. None of these.

20.6 Extrapyramidal effects include
   A. Dystonia.
   B. Parkinsonian signs and symptoms.
   C. Tardive dyskinesia.
   D. All of these.
   E. None of these.

20.7 Medications that can improve the akathisia produced by high-potency neuroleptics are
   A. Benzodiazepines and beta-blockers.
   B. Tricyclic antidepressants (TCAs) and monoamine oxidase inhibitors (MAOIs).
   C. Lithium and carbamazepine.
   D. All of these.
   E. None of these.

20.8 Agranulocytosis is a rare complication of neuroleptic medication and
   A. Is most likely to occur in the first few months of treatment.
   B. Is most likely to occur after 12 months of treatment.
   C. Is most likely to occur after 24 months of treatment.
   D. All of these.
   E. None of these.

Pharmacological Treatment

20.9 The mortality rate among persons with neuroleptic malignant syndrome is
   A. 10%.
   B. 20%.
   C. 30%.
   D. All of these.
   E. None of these.

20.10 Catatonia caused by neuroleptic medication presents with
   A. Rigidity.
   B. Immobility.
   C. Waxy flexibility.
   D. All of these.
   E. None of these.

20.11 Secondary amines are produced from tertiary amines by
   A. The addition of a methyl group.
   B. The deletion of a methyl group.
   C. The conversion of a methyl group into a sulfonylurea group.
   D. All of these.
   E. None of these.

20.12 The rate of seizure associated with treatment with a TCA is
   A. 1 in 100,000.
   B. 1 in 10,000.
   C. 1 in 1,000.
   D. All of these.
   E. None of these.

20.13 TCA act as type 1 quinidine-like antiarrhythmic agents resulting in
   A. An increased PR interval on electrocardiogram (ECG).
   B. An increased QRS interval on ECG.
   C. An increased QT interval on ECG.
   D. All of these.
   E. None of these.

20.14 In patients with normal cardiac function, imipramine and nortriptyline have an incidence of 2:1 block of
A. 0.7%.
B. 0.9%.
C. 1%.
D. All of these.
E. None of these.

20.15 Treatment of a major depressive disorder with a TCA should continue for a minimum of
A. 12 months.
B. 6 months.
C. 3 months.
D. All of these.
E. None of these.

20.16 The average length of an untreated major depressive episode in a person over age 50 is
A. 1–2 years.
B. 3–5 years.
C. 6–7 years.
D. All of these.
E. None of these.

20.17 MAOIs are grouped as hydrazine and nonhydrazine types and have the following characteristics
A. Hydrazine MAOIs (e.g., phenelzine) are more hepatotoxic.
B. Efficacy between hydrazine and nonhydrazine MAOIs differs.
C. Both hydrazine and nonhydrazine MAOIs are reversible inhibitors of monoamine oxidase enzymes.
D. All of these.
E. None of these.

20.18 Patients taking an MAOI who use a pressor agent (e.g., pseudoephedrine) may experience a hypertensive crisis. The incidence of hypertensive crises may be as high as
A. 4%.
B. 6%.
C. 8%.
D. All of these.
E. None of these.

Pharmacological Treatment

20.19 A critical determinant of outcome with MAOI therapy is
   A. Dose.
   B. Compliance.
   C. Use of hydrazine versus nonhydrazine.
   D. All of these.
   E. None of these.

20.20 Fluoxetine, a selective serotonin reuptake inhibitor (SSRI) has the following characteristics
   A. It has a metabolite with a long half-life (norfluoxetine).
   B. It significantly potentiates TCAs and some benzodiazepines.
   C. It induces weight loss and anorexia in the elderly.
   D. All of these.
   E. None of these.

20.21 Buproprion is an aminoketone antidepressant that
   A. Can cause hypotension and conduction changes.
   B. Has a risk of seizures with doses of 450 mg or higher.
   C. Needs to be administered three times per day.
   D. All of these.
   E. None of these.

20.22 Alprazolam
   A. Has an antidepressant effect.
   B. Lacks a cardiovascular or autonomic effect.
   C. Produces sedation and withdrawal seizures.
   D. All of these.
   E. None of these.

20.23 When a stimulant trial is initiated,
   A. A rapid response should occur within 3 days if effective.
   B. There should be a concern about the potential for abuse and dependence.
   C. Improvement occurs in mood, motivation, and psychomotor state if the trial is effective.
   D. All of these.
   E. None of these.

20.24 Plasma level for nonacute lithium prophylaxis in the elderly should be
   A. 0.4–0.7 mmol/L.
   B. 1.0–1.4 mmol/L.
   C. 3.0–3.5 mmol/L.
   D. All of these.
   E. None of these.

20.25 Carbamazepine levels may be increased by the concomitant use of
   A. Propoxyphene.
   B. Diltiazem and verapamil.
   C. Erythromycin.
   D. All of these.
   E. None of these.

20.26 Oxazepam and lorazepam
   A. Are metabolized by conjugation.
   B. Do not yield active metabolites.
   C. Are less likely to produce cumulative side effects.
   D. All of these.
   E. None of these.

20.27 The percentage of neuroleptic-treated patients who develop extrapyramidal side effects (EPS) is
   A. 10%–20%.
   B. 20%–40%.
   C. 40%–60%.
   D. All of these.
   E. None of these.

20.28 In prescribing medication in the elderly, it is important
   A. To begin with low doses.
   B. To increase slowly.
   C. To monitor for symptom change and the emergence of side effects.
   D. All of these.
   E. None of these.

Pharmacological Treatment

Directions: For each of the statements below, one or more of the answers is correct. Choose

- A. If 1, 2, and 3 are correct.
- B. If only 1 and 3 are correct.
- C. If only 2 and 4 are correct.
- D. If only 4 is correct.
- E. If all are correct.

20.29 The processes involved in drug disposition include
1. Absorption.
2. Distribution.
3. Metabolism.
4. Elimination.

20.30 Lipophilic medications that may increase in the elderly include
1. Antidepressants.
2. Antipsychotics.
3. Benzodiazepines.
4. Lithium.

20.31 Factors affecting drug distribution in the elderly include
1. Decline in total body water.
2. Increase in cardiac output.
3. Decrease in serum albumin.
4. Increase in renal clearance.

20.32 Factors to consider when initiating antipsychotic medication include
1. Adequacy of hydration.
2. Degree of orthostasis.
3. Cardiac function.
4. Concomitant medications.

20.33 High-potency neuroleptics
1. Are long acting.
2. Are less sedating.
3. Produce orthostasis.
4. Induce extrapyramidal reactions.

20.34 Low-potency neuroleptics are more likely to produce
1. Conduction changes.
2. Ventricular arrhythmias.
3. Torsade de pointes.
4. Atrial arrhythmias.

20.35 Liquid preparations of neuroleptic medication are advantageous when
1. Compliance is questioned.
2. EPS are present.
3. Swallowing pills or a capsule is a problem.
4. The patient is agitated.

20.36 In the elderly, doses of medication should be prescribed
1. At 85% of the suggested adult dose.
2. At 75% of the suggested adult dose.
3. At 65% of the suggested adult dose.
4. At 50% of the suggested adult dose.

20.37 Factors to consider in initiating antidepressant medication include checking for
1. History of prior treatment.
2. Family history of treatment for depression.
3. Clarification of all current medications being taken.
4. The use of alcohol and other drugs.

20.38 Older patients with a depressive disorder nonresponsive or partially responsive to TCA may require augmentation with
1. Lithium.
2. Triiodothyronine.
3. SSRIs.
4. Tryptophane.

20.39 Anticholinergic effects are more pronounced when MAOIs are used with
1. TCAs.
2. Antihistamines.
3. Antiparkinsonian drugs.
4. Lithium.

Pharmacological Treatment 141

20.40 Orthostatic and lying systolic blood pressure may drop in older patients treated with MAOIs. Symptoms reported include
1. Dizziness.
2. Weakness.
3. Inability to stand up.
4. No complaints.

20.41 Tranylcypromine compared with phenelzine is more likely to cause
1. Anorexia and weight loss.
2. Agitation.
3. Headache.
4. Insomnia.

20.42 SSRIs
1. Are free of cardiovascular and autonomic side effects associated with MAOIs and TCAs.
2. Interact with valproic acid, phenelzine, buspirone, and neuroleptics.
3. Potentiate the effects of TCAs and benzodiazepines.
4. Have become first- and second-line treatments for depression.

20.43 Indications for the use of stimulants include use in
1. Medically ill patients with depression.
2. Patients with withdrawn postoperative states.
3. Patients who have poststroke depression.
4. Patients with anxiety states.

20.44 Benign side effects of lithium therapy include
1. Fine tremor.
2. Headache and nausea.
3. Tiredness.
4. Polyuria.

20.45 Petit mal status is seen with
1. Carbamazepine and diltiazem.
2. Lithium and TCA.
3. Methylphenidate and TCA.
4. Valproate and clonazepam.

20.46 The effect of benzodiazepine is potentiated by
1. Alcohol.
2. MAOIs.
3. Sedating TCAs.
4. Antihypertensives.

20.47 Benzodiazepines are indicated in the treatment of
1. Generalized anxiety disorder.
2. Posttraumatic stress disorder.
3. Panic disorder.
4. Alcohol withdrawal.

20.48 Classes of medications effective in the treatment of neuroleptic-induced EPS include
1. Anticholinergics.
2. Antihistamines.
3. Beta-blockers.
4. Benzodiazepines.

20.49 Ergoloid mesylates in doses of up to 7.5 mg/day for 12 weeks were found to
1. Reduce confusion.
2. Reduce recent memory impairment.
3. Reduce depression.
4. Reduce emotional lability.

20.50 Indications for the use of intramuscular or intravenous neuroleptic medications include
1. Agitation and combativeness in a patient with organic brain syndrome.
2. Acute psychosis in a debilitated elderly person.
3. A very agitated intensive care patient.
4. An acutely bereaved elderly person.

ANSWERS

20.1 The answer is **D**. Older persons taking multiple medications are at an increased risk to have problems with compliance, to experience drug-

Pharmacological Treatment 143

drug interactions, and to experience physician-caused (iatrogenic) illness **(p. 359)**.

20.2 The answer is **D**. Medications that are excreted by the kidney are affected by the age-related decline in renal function and perfusion, which can result in higher serum levels for a given dose of medication. Specific psychoactive medications excreted by the kidneys include lithium, dextroamphetamine, fluvoxamine, and nortriptyline **(p. 360)**.

20.3 The answer is **B**. As the person with early-onset schizophrenia ages, the person exhibits withdrawal in contrast to the agitation and frank hallucinations of earlier years **(p. 361)**.

20.4 The answer is **B**. The aliphatic phenothiazines are examples of low-potency neuroleptics and are nonspecific in their effects. They affect other systems besides the dopaminergic system, producing marked anticholinergic, antiadrenergic, and sedative effects **(p. 361)**

20.5 The answer is **B**. Piperidine phenothiazines are preferred in the elderly because of their sedative properties **(p. 361)**. Tertiary antidepressants are converted to secondary amines by demethylation. These secondary amines are better tolerated in the elderly because of their lower side-effect profile **(p. 364)**.

20.6 The answer is **D**. Extrapyramidal effects seen with high-potency neuroleptics include dystonia, Parkinsonian symptoms (tremor, rigidity, and rabbit syndrome), akathisia, akinesia, and tardive dyskinesia **(p. 362)**.

20.7 The answer is **A**. Benzodiazepines and beta-blockers have been found to be helpful with akathisia **(p. 362)**.

20.8 The answer is **A**. Agranulocytosis is a rare complication of neuroleptic medication occurring in approximately 1 in 100,000 people treated with neuroleptics. It occurs within the first few months of treatment. Seventy-five percent of all cases of agranulocytosis occur in persons age 50 and older **(p. 363)**.

20.9 The answer is **B**. The mortality rate among persons with neuroleptic malignant syndrome is 20% **(p. 363)**.

20.10 The answer is **D**. Catatonia resulting from the use of neuroleptic medications presents with rigidity, immobility, and waxy flexibility. Antiparkinsonian medication is ineffective in its treatment **(p. 363)**.

20.11 The answer is **B**. Removing a methyl group from a tertiary amine produces a secondary amine TCA that is better tolerated by the elderly **(p. 364)**.

20.12 The answer is **C**. The risk of seizure with TCA is 1 in 1,000 and can be as a high as 3 in 100 if high doses of imipramine are used in a patient with atypical depression **(p. 365)**.

20.13 The answer is **D**. The change in the ECG seen with the use of TCA include increases in the PR, QRS, and QT intervals **(p. 366)**.

20.14 The answer is **A**. In older patients, with normal medical cardiac function, the incidence of 2:1 atrioventricular block is 0.7% for nortriptyline **(p. 366)**.

20.15 The answer is **B**. The treatment of a major depressive episode should continue for a minimum of 6 months **(p. 367)**. The recent Practice Guidelines of the American Psychiatric Association recommend treatment for 9 months.

20.16 The answer is **B**. An untreated episode of depression in a person over age 50 lasts an average of 3–5 years. For a person age 31–50 years, the natural course of an untreated depressive episode is 9–18 months **(p. 367)**.

20.17 The answer is **A**. Hydrazine type MAOIs (phenelzine) are purportedly more hepatotoxic than nonhydrazine MAOIs (tranylcypromine and deprenyl). But the risk is exceedingly low. There is no overall difference in efficacy between the types of MAOIs. Both hydrazine and nonhydrazine MAOIs are irreversible inhibitors of the monoamine oxidase enzyme inactivating the available supply of the enzyme. It requires 10–14 days for the body's synthesis of new monoamine oxidase enzyme to bring levels back to normal **(pp. 367–368)**.

20.18 The answer is **C**. The incidence of hypertensive crisis in patients taking an MAOI may be as high as 8%. Pressure agents that may prompt a hypertensive crisis include tyramine, phenylephedrine, phenylpropanolamine, pseudoephedrine, amphetamine **(p. 368)**.

20.19 The answer is **A**. A critical determinant of outcome in MAOI therapy is dose. An increase of 15 mg of phenelzine, 5 mg of isocarboxazide, or 10 mg of tranylcypromine may be pivotal in response versus nonresponse **(p. 369)**.

20.20 The answer is **E**. Fluoxetine, an SSRI, has an active metabolite (norfluoxetine) with a very long half-life. Fluoxetine potentiates the

Pharmacological Treatment

effects of TCA and some benzodiazepines and can induce weight loss in the elderly (p. 369).

20.21 The answer is **A**. Buproprion is a nonserotinergic antidepressant that is well tolerated in the elderly and produced minimal hypotension and conduction changes. It does have a risk of seizures at high does of 450 mg and above. Its principle drawback is the need for administration three times per day at the upper dosage range of 400–450 mg/day (p. 369).

20.22 The answer is **D**. Alprazolam has antianxiety and antidepressant effects. It does not have the autonomic and cardiovascular effects of TCA. Seizures have been reported with abrupt withdrawal of alprazolam (p. 370).

20.23 The answer is **D**. The use of stimulants (dextroamphetamine and methylphenidate) is characterized by rapid onset of response—within 3 days, if effective. Reservations about using stimulant medication have related to the concern about the potential for abuse or dependence. If the trial of a stimulant is successful, improvement in mood, motivation, psychomotor state, sleep, and appetite are noted (p. 370).

20.24 The answer is **A**. For nonacute elderly patients on lithium prophylaxis, lithium levels should range between 0.4–0.7 mmol/L (p. 371).

20.25 The answer is **C**. Concurrent use of propoxyphene, diltiazem, verapamil, and erythromycin increase the blood level of carbamazepine (p. 372).

20.26 The answer is **D**. Oxazepam and lorazepam, short-acting benzodiazepines, are metabolized by conjugation and do not have active metabolites. They are less likely to produce cumulative sedation (p. 373).

20.27 The answer is **B**. Some 20%–40% of patients treated with neuroleptics will develop EPS (p. 375).

20.28 The answer is **B**. When prescribing medication in the elderly, it is important to begin with a low dose, to increase the medication slowly, and to monitor the patient for changes in symptoms with treatment and for the emergence of side effects (p. 377).

20.29 The answer is **E**. The four main processes involved in drug disposition are absorption, distribution, metabolism, and elimination (p. 360).

20.30 The answer is **A**. With aging, the percentage of total body fat increases resulting in a large volume of distribution for lipophilic drugs, medications stored in fatty tissues. Psychoactive medications that are lipophilic include antidepressants, antipsychotics, and benzodiazepines **(p. 360)**.

20.31 The answer is **B**. Drug disposition in the elderly is affected by the age-related physiologic changes of aging, which include an increase in total body fat (25%–45%), a decline in total body water, a decrease in serum albumin (as much as 25%), and a decline in renal function and perfusion **(p. 360)**.

20.32 The answer is **E**. When initiating treatment with a neuroleptic, several factors must be considered: the patient's age, adequacy of hydration, degree of orthostasis, cardiac function, concomitant medications, and severity of psychotic symptoms **(p. 361)**.

20.33 The answer is **C**. High-potency neuroleptics are less sedating and induce extrapyramidal reactions but do not produce orthostasis **(p. 362)**.

20.34 The answer is **A**. Low-potency neuroleptics can produce conductive changes and ventricular arrhythmias including torsade de pointes **(p. 363)**.

20.35 The answer is **B**. Liquid preparations of neuroleptic medications are useful when compliance is a question and when swallowing pills or capsules is a problem **(p. 363)**.

20.36 The answer is **D**. Due to the physiologic changes of aging, the initiation of treatment with a dose of no more than 50% of the recommended adult does should be done. The dose should be increased slowly **(p. 360)**.

20.37 The answer is **A**. When selecting an antidepressant, it is important to check for a history of prior treatment and to establish whether a family member has been treated for depression (with which medication and with what response). Current medications being taken should be clarified, and the patient's use of alcohol and other drugs should be determined as well **(p. 364)**.

20.38 The answer is **A**. An older person with a major depressive disorder that is nonresponsive or partially responsive to a TCA may have medications added to the TCA to augment its effect. Medications used in augmentation include lithium, with which it may take 3–4 weeks to

Pharmacological Treatment

show improvement. Triiodothyronine (25 µg) may be added to a TCA to augments its effect. SSRI may be added, also, to potentiate the effects of a partial TCA response **(p. 367)**.

20.39 The answer is **A**. When MAOIs are used with TCA, antihistamines, or antiparkinsonian drugs, anticholinergic effects are more pronounced. Impaired sexual arousal, constipation, and urinary delay (hesitancy), are less with MAOIs at low doses but may become a concern with combined treatments **(p. 368)**.

20.40 The answer is **E**. Although orthostatic blood pressure changes may be associated with complaints of dizziness, weakness, and inability to stand up, these blood pressure changes may be asymptomatic and may not occur until 3 weeks of treatment **(p. 368)**.

20.41 The answer is **E**. Tranylcypromine (nonhydrazine MAOI) compared with phenelzine (hydrazine MAOI) is more likely to cause anorexia, weight loss, agitation, headache, and insomnia. Weight gain, myoclonus, and memory impairment are the side effects usually reported for MAOIs **(p. 368)**.

20.42 The answer is **E**. SSRIs are free of the autonomic and cardiovascular side effects of TCA and MAOIs. Interactions with valproic acid, phenelzine, buspirone, and neuroleptics need to be monitored. Fluoxetine, sertraline, and paroxetine have become the first and second choices in initiating treatment for a major depressive disorder in the elderly because of the efficacy and safety of these SSRIs **(p. 369)**.

20.43 The answer is **A**. Stimulants have been shown to be effective in medically ill patients with depression, in patients with postoperative states, and in patients who have poststroke depression **(p. 370)**.

20.44 The answer is **E**. Fine tremor, nausea, tiredness, and polyurea are benign side effects of lithium therapy. Other side effects include weight gain, thyroid enlargement, hypothyroidism, diabetes insipidus, psoriasis, skin infection, and sinus arrhythmias **(p. 371)**.

20.45 The answer is **D**. The combination of valproate and clonazepam can lead to petit mal status **(p. 373)**.

20.46 The answer is **E**. Benzodiazepines used with alcohol, MAOIs, neuroleptics, and antihypertensive medications have their effects potentiated **(p. 373)**.

20.47 The answer is **E**. Benzodiazepines are indicated in the treatment of generalized anxiety disorder, posttraumatic stress disorder, panic disorder, acute states of anxiety and agitation, and alcohol withdrawal **(p. 373)**.

20.48 The answer is **E**. Anticholinergics, antihistamines, beta-blockers, and benzodiazepines are all effective in treating neuroleptic-induced EPS **(p. 375)**.

20.49 The answer is **E**. Ergoloid mesylates (hydergine) administered over 12 weeks improved confusion, recent memory impairment, depression, and emotional lability **(p. 376)**.

20.50 The answer is **A**. Indications for the use of intramuscular or intravenous medication include agitation and combativeness in older persons with organic brain syndromes, an acutely psychotic debilitated older person, and the very agitated intensive care patient. Very low doses of 0.5 mg of haloperidol are injected 2 or 3 times per day as an initial approach to providing symptomatic relief **(p. 363)**.

CHAPTER 21

Diet, Nutrition, and Exercise

QUESTIONS

Directions: **Select the single best response for each of the following questions.**

21.1 Age-related factors affecting diet include all except
   A. Deterioration in taste buds and olfactory sensation.
   B. Onset of illness.
   C. Pattern of increased exercise.
   D. All of these.
   E. None of these.

21.2 The science of nutrition is defined as
   A. The study of nutrients, nutrition, and biomass.
   B. The study of food intake to promote growth and to replace injured tissue.
   C. The study of metabolism, calorie utilization, and trace element utilization.
   D. All of these.
   E. None of these.

21.3 Change in height in the elderly is due to
   A. Vertebral compression fractures.
   B. Kyphosis.
   C. Spinal disc collapse.
   D. All of these.
   E. None of these.

21.4 The most clinically practical and cost-effective way to determine body fat stores is to
   A. Weigh the patient.
   B. Fluid-restrict the patient, then weigh the patient.
   C. Use calipers to measure skin-fold thickness.
   D. All of these.
   E. None of these.

21.5 A lymphocyte count of below 1,500/mL is
   A. Evidence of an inadequate diet.
   B. Evidence of an infection.
   C. Evidence of depleted fat stores.
   D. All of these.
   E. None of these.

21.6 Malnourishment among surgical patients was found to be
   A. 5%–20%.
   B. 15%–30%.
   C. 30%–65%.
   D. All of these.
   E. None of these.

21.7 Symptoms of lactase deficiency include
   A. Uncomfortable gas production.
   B. Diarrhea.
   C. Cramping 1–2 hours after eating dairy products.
   D. All of these.
   E. None of these.

21.8 An important factor for diabetics who are insulin resistant is
   A. Achieving ideal weight.
   B. Taking a daily walk.
   C. Increasing protein consumption.
   D. All of these.
   E. None of these.

Diet, Nutrition, and Exercise

21.9 Vitamin C used in excess may have toxic effects because of its potential to
   A. Create renal oxalate stones.
   B. Produce diarrhea.
   C. Interfere with B_{12} absorption.
   D. All of these.
   E. None of these.

Directions: **For each of the statements below, one or more of the answers is correct. Choose**

   A. If 1, 2, and 3 are correct.
   B. If only 1 and 3 are correct.
   C. If only 2 and 4 are correct.
   D. If only 4 is correct.
   E. If all are correct.

21.10 Techniques used to measure body fat stores include
   1. Bioelectric impedance.
   2. Tritium dilution.
   3. Dual-photon absorptiometry.
   4. Water immersion.

21.11 Weight loss can result from
   1. Depression.
   2. Dementia.
   3. Congestive heart failure.
   4. Chronic infection.

21.12 Dietary fiber may prevent cancer by
   1. Reducing intraluminal colon pressure.
   2. Decreasing fecal transit time.
   3. Binding noxious agents (deoxycholic acid and lithocholic acid).
   4. Decreasing the amount of nitrosamines.

21.13 Patients who have had a stroke may be unable to eat because of
   1. Paralysis.
   2. Confusion.
   3. Unconsciousness.
   4. Respiratory problems.

21.14 The elements of an exercise program include
1. Flexibility.
2. Strength.
3. Endurance.
4. Oxygen saturation.

21.15 The components necessary to improve endurance include
1. A focus on aerobic conditioning.
2. The ability of the respiratory system to respond to the demands of exercise.
3. The ability of the cardiovascular system to respond to extended periods of muscle activity without fatigue.
4. Increased strength.

ANSWERS

21.1 The answer is **C**. Exercise habits can be taken for granted. The gradual reduction in physical activity in late life is associated with a reduction in appetite. Changes in living habits associated with retirement, the onset of illness, and deterioration in taste buds and olfactory sensation combine to create special dietary demands and change prior dietary patterns **(p. 381)**.

21.2 The answer is **B**. The science of nutrition is defined as the study of food intake to promote growth and to replace worn or injured tissue **(p. 381)**.

21.3 The answer is **D**. Changes in the height of older adults have several causes. Vertebral compression fractures, kyphosis, and spinal disc collapse contribute to changes in height in the elderly **(p. 381)**.

21.4 The answer is **C**. Measurement of skin-fold thickness by caliper remains the daily, clinical standard for determining body fat stores **(p. 382)**.

21.5 The answer is **A**. A useful indicator of an inadequate diet is a lymphocyte count below 1,500/mL **(p. 382)**.

21.6 The answer is **C**. Between 30% and 65% of surgical patients were found to be malnourished. Some 17%–44% of medical patients were found to be malnourished **(p. 382)**.

Diet, Nutrition, and Exercise

21.7 The answer is **D**. Lactase deficiency results in uncomfortable symptoms of gas production, diarrhea, and cramping within 1–2 hours of eating dairy products **(p. 385)**.

21.8 The answer is **A**. Insulin-resistant diabetics will benefit the most from achieving an ideal weight through a reduction of total calories **(p. 385)**.

21.9 The answer is **D**. Because of its effect on immune mechanisms, the inhibition of nitrosamine formation in the stomach, and antioxidative effects, vitamin C may be protective in the aging process. Overuse of vitamin C can produce toxic effects including the creation of renal oxalate stones, the production of diarrhea, and interference with vitamin B_{12} absorption **(p. 387)**.

21.10 The answer is **E**. Body fat stores are the energy reserves of the body. Accurate water immersion studies are difficult and time consuming. Newer techniques that are technically interesting for research studies include bioelectric impedance, tritium dilution, and dual-photon absorptiometry **(p. 382)**.

21.11 The answer is **E**. Although the underlying mechanism modulating appetite needs to be clarified several illnesses have been found to decrease appetite: congestive heart failure, lung failure, renal failure, chronic infection, depression, and dementia **(p. 382)**.

21.12 The answer is **B**. Dietary fiber prevents cancer by several mechanisms. Transit time of fecal material in the gut is speeded up, decreasing the amount of gut contact time. Deoxycholic acid and lithocholic acid, noxious elements, are bound by dietary fiber **(p. 384)**.

21.13 The answer is **A**. Patients who have had a stroke may be unable to eat because of paralysis, confusion, or unconsciousness **(p. 386)**.

21.14 The answer is **A**. The three key components of an exercise program involve flexibility, strength, and endurance **(p. 389)**.

21.15 The answer is **A**. Aerobic exercise is a form of training that will enhance the cardiovascular system to improve its endurance. This training requires the individual to stay within limits that permit inhaled oxygen to fully supply the body's needs during exercise by increasing the efficiency of oxygen transport and use from the lungs to each cell. Improved oxygen use permits extended periods of muscle activity without fatigue **(p. 389)**.

CHAPTER 22

Psychotherapy

QUESTIONS

Directions: **Select the single best response for each of the following questions.**

22.1 Risks to the elderly mind include
   A. Prescription drug and alcohol abuse.
   B. Dementia and depression.
   C. Maladaptive emotional response to predictable crises of late life.
   D. All of these.
   E. None of these.

22.2 The treatment of depression based on the recommendations of the Consensus Development Panel on Depression in Late Life recommended
   A. The exclusive use of psychosocial intervention for the treatment of depression.
   B. Insight-oriented psychoanalysis for the treatment of depression.
   C. The exclusive use of cognitive-behavior therapy.
   D. All of these.
   E. None of these.

22.3 Freud believed that the elderly were not good candidates for psychotherapy because the elderly
   A. Lacked the elasticity of mind needed for psychotherapy.
   B. Had so much material in their long lives to deal with that the analysis would be unmanageable in time.
   C. Lacked sufficient life span to benefit from the analysis.
   D. All of these.
   E. None of these.

22.4 An important resource describing the emotional life of an octogenarian was written by an analytic psychologist named
   A. Eric Abraham.
   B. Florida Scott-Maxwell.
   C. George Caisson-Stewart.
   D. All of these.
   E. None of these.

22.5 The psychological issues in late life described by Erickson included
   A. Personality development in the eighth stage of life with resolution of the conflict between ego integrity and despair.
   B. The "afternoon" and "evening" of life—a time of opportunity to shift toward growth as a mature individual.
   C. A continuing struggle to maintain self-esteem with increasing narcissistic threat and loss.
   D. All of these.
   E. None of these.

22.6 Social science theory has suggested that the replacement of social roles and relationships is the important task across the life span. This is termed the
   A. *Disengagement theory.*
   B. *Activity theory.*
   C. *Continuity theory.*
   D. All of these.
   E. None of these.

22.7 In Freidan's confrontation of the "age mystique," she suggests that old age should be viewed
   A. As a unique story of life.
   B. A stage of life with its own pattern of relationships, career, sex, and family.
   C. Not as a stage of deterioration, decline, and loss.
   D. All of these.
   E. None of these.

22.8 Factors considered in the clinician's decision to use insight-oriented versus supportive psychotherapy include
   A. The patient's age.
   B. The patient's gender.
   C. The patient's past and current capacity for object relatedness.
   D. All of these.
   E. None of these.

22.9 Supportive psychotherapy has emphasized the assessment of ego functioning and the restraint required for psychotherapy. It
   A. Provides reassurance for the elderly patient.
   B. Increases semantic complaints.
   C. Rarely uses psychoeducational components.
   D. All of these.
   E. None of these.

22.10 A study of the process and outcome of brief psychodynamic psychotherapy found that
   A. The therapist was used to validate normalcy.
   B. The therapist was used to validate competency.
   C. The therapist was used to aid in the restoration of a positive sense of self.
   D. All of these.
   E. None of these.

22.11 Based on the published literatures, the overall efficacy of brief dynamic psychotherapy was
   A. 55%.
   B. 45%.
   C. 35%.
   D. All of these.
   E. None of these.

22.12 Cognitive-behavior therapy is
   A. Open ended.
   B. Exploratory.
   C. Developed for use in patients with schizoid and anxiety disorders.
   D. All of these.
   E. None of these.

22.13 Interpersonal therapy began with the work of
  A. Freud.
  B. Jung.
  C. Sullivan.
  D. All of these.
  E. None of these.

22.14 In interpersonal psychotherapy, the role of the therapist is
  A. Teacher.
  B. Patient advocate.
  C. Critic.
  D. All of these.
  E. None of these.

22.15 *Life review* is defined as
  A. A universal mental process of the elderly as they confront the myths of their invulnerability or immortality.
  B. Composed of four primary constructs described by Viney.
  C. An atypical development stage.
  D. All of these.
  E. None of these.

22.16 Existential psychotherapy is
  A. A specific psychodynamic therapeutic approach.
  B. A method of exploration in psychotherapy.
  C. An extension of reminiscence.
  D. All of these.
  E. None of these.

22.17 Group psychotherapy in institutions can
  A. Halt regression.
  B. Facilitate reengagement.
  C. Encourage problem solving.
  D. All of these.
  E. None of these.

22.18 Examples of issue- or problem-focused support or self-help groups include
   A. Retirement adjustment groups.
   B. Widowhood groups.
   C. Caregivers groups for caregivers of Alzheimer's patients.
   D. All of these.
   E. None of these.

Directions: **For each of the statements below, one or more of the answers is correct. Choose**

   A. If 1, 2, and 3 are correct.
   B. If only 1 and 3 are correct.
   C. If only 2 and 4 are correct.
   D. If only 4 is correct.
   E. If all are correct.

22.19 Trends affecting the treatment of psychiatric disorder in the elderly include
   1. An increase in scientific knowledge.
   2. The rapidly changing health care system.
   3. An emphasis upon outcome.
   4. The cost-effectiveness of care.

22.20 Age-related barriers to psychotherapy have been reported as
   1. The belief that older persons have a decreased capacity for abstraction and new learning.
   2. The perception that defenses and personality characteristics are fixed and immutable.
   3. The recognition of the limitations in internal and external resources and choices for the elderly.
   4. The absence of psychological mindedness in the elderly.

22.21 Spirituality is important in late life because it
   1. Suggests strategies for growth.
   2. Emphasizes that the individual must grow and learn.
   3. Results in empowerment.
   4. Notes that old age may be viewed as a unique phase in the life cycle.

22.22 Barriers to psychotherapy in the elderly include
1. The family's perception that psychiatric symptoms are a normal part of aging.
2. The negative attitude of therapists toward the elderly.
3. The inadequacy of medicine and other third-party reimbursement for therapy.
4. The belief that psychiatric symptoms relate to medical illness and the assumption that they are untreatable.

22.23 The countertransference that may be experienced by the younger therapist treating the older patient includes
1. Unconscious hostility due to anger with one's parents.
2. Increased expectation of the elder because of the elder's life experiences.
3. Avoidance of conflictual material due to deferential respect for the patient.
4. Anticipation of an erotic countertransference.

22.24 Because they anticipate a shorter life span, older persons frequently have
1. A decreased resistance to change.
2. An increased resistance to change.
3. Increased motivation for therapy.
4. Decreased motivation for therapy.

22.25 The goals of brief (time-limited) dynamic psychotherapy are
1. To obtain symptomatic relief.
2. To achieve insight into behavioral patterns.
3. To enhance self-esteem.
4. To complete structural characterological change.

22.26 When older men and women were compared concerning the outcome of brief psychodynamic psychotherapy,
1. Women were found to show improvement earlier.
2. Men were found to show improvement earlier.
3. Women maintained their improvement longer.
4. Men maintained their improvement longer.

Psychotherapy **161**

22.27 When treating elderly depressed patients with cognitive-behavior therapy, the therapy must
   1. Socialize the older person to the treatment process.
   2. Recognize the potential presence of hearing or visual deficits.
   3. Utilize examples specific to the older person's age.
   4. Acknowledge the older person's expectation of significant benefit from psychotherapy.

22.28 The behavioral treatment of depression emphasizes the learning of social skills by
   1. Time management.
   2. Assertiveness training.
   3. Improving cognitive skills to decrease negative thought.
   4. Improving social/communication skills.

22.29 Interpersonal therapy is characterized as
   1. Long term.
   2. Focused.
   3. Emphasizing past relationships.
   4. Interpersonal.

22.30 Factors identified as linked to therapeutic effectiveness or change in group therapy include
   1. Instillation of hope.
   2. Universality and altruism.
   3. Corrective recapitulation of the primary family group.
   4. Interpersonal learning.

22.31 Specific forms of psychotherapy used in group psychotherapy include
   1. Psychodynamic.
   2. Interpersonal.
   3. Supportive.
   4. Cognitive behavior.

22.32 Combined treatment, psychotherapy, and pharmacotherapy
1. Are contraindicated because medications interfere with the psychodynamic process.
2. Are indicated for patients with more severe depression with associated melancholia.
3. Are only useful after 16 weeks of psychotherapy with only a partial response.
4. Are indicated in patients who have had only a partial response to either treatment alone.

22.33 Factors to consider in treating old patients include
1. Providing seating of adequate height with a firm seat.
2. Providing lighting sufficient in intensity.
3. Using written material with large type.
4. Addressing the patient by the patient's surname.

ANSWERS

22.1 The answer is **D**. Fogel et al. identified seven major risks to the elderly mind: dementia, depression, schizophrenia and other chronic mental illnesses, behavioral and emotional consequences of nondementing brain disease, prescription drug and alcohol abuse, maladaptive emotional responses to predictable crises of late life, and prescription drug psychotoxicity **(p. 395)**.

22.2 The answer is **E**. The Consensus Development Panel on Depression in Late Life concluded that cognitive-behavior therapy, interpersonal therapy, and short-term dynamic therapy constitute the recommended psychotherapeutic interventions for the treatment of the depressed elderly. Although psychosocial interventions were considered an important part of treatment in this population, they were not recommended as the exclusive treatment. The report recommended marital and family interventions as well as community-based psychosocial interventions as indicated **(pp. 395–396)**.

22.3 The answer is **D**. Although he continued his own analysis to age 83, Freud believed that the elderly were not good psychotherapeutic candidates for psychoanalysis. He believed that the elderly lacked the elasticity of mind necessary for psychotherapy and would require an unmeasurable length of time to go through their long life histories. He

Psychotherapy

was also skeptical of the long-term benefits and economic value of psychoanalysis for the elderly **(p. 396)**.

22.4 The answer is **B**. Florida Scott-Maxwell, an analytic psychologist, provided a vivid account of her emotional life as an octogenarian. She described her life in her 80s in the journal *The Measure of My Days* **(p. 396)**.

22.5 The answer is **A**. Erickson focused on late life or the eighth stage of psychological development. He described this stage of life as characterized by the resolution of the conflict between ego integrity and ego despair resulting in ego integrity. Jung described the latter part of the life cycle as the "afternoon" and "evening" of life, a time of opportunities with a shift from the emphasis on work, family, and societal involvement (outward focus) to mature individuation (inward focus) **(p. 397)**.

22.6 The answer is **B**. There are three divergent social science theories concerning the best way to conceptualize aging. The *activity theory* suggests the importance of replacing social roles and relationships with new roles and relationships as transition occurs across the life span. The *continuity theory* suggests that the pattern of social involvement characteristic of earlier life remain unchanged. In contrast, the *disengagement theory* stresses the gradual withdrawal from social roles, which is beneficial to the individual and society **(p. 397)**.

22.7 The answer is **D**. Challenging the concept of old age as a time of deterioration, decline, and loss, Freidan suggests that late life be viewed as a unique stage of life with its own patterns for relationships, career, sex, family, and involvement—a time of potential growth **(p. 397)**.

22.8 The answer is **C**. The clinician decision to emphasize insight versus supportive work is based on information obtained in the initial assessment. The patient's history of current and past object relationships, degree of psychological mindedness, and depth of motivation to change are valuable data aiding the clinician's decision **(p. 399)**.

22.9 The answer is **A**. Emphasizing the assessment of ego functioning and the restraint necessary for supportive psychotherapy, this form of individual psychotherapy provides reassurance for the elderly patient and attempts to decrease anxiety and enhance the person's feeling of self worth. Somatic complaints may be reduced as their causes are identified. Psychoeducational components may be used to enhance the older person's ego strength **(p. 399)**.

22.10 The answer is **D**. In one study of the process and outcome of brief psychodynamic psychotherapy, the therapist was used to validate normalcy and competency and to assist in restoration of a positive sense of self **(p. 400)**.

22.11 The answer is **C**. Based on a literature review, the American Psychiatric Association Task Force on Models of Practice in Geriatric Psychiatry found the overall efficacy of brief dynamic psychotherapy to be 35% **(p. 400)**.

22.12 The answer is **E**. *Cognitive-behavior therapy* is defined as a time-limited, focused psychotherapy. It was developed for use in patients with depression **(p. 400)**.

22.13 The answer is **E**. Recognizing the important role of social relationship, Harry Stack Sullivan developed a form of psychotherapy that focused on social relationships throughout the life cycle termed *interpersonal psychotherapy* **(p. 401)**.

22.14 The answer is **B**. In interpersonal psychotherapy, the therapist role is that of patient advocate, being nonjudgmental while communicating warmth and unconditional positive regard **(p. 402)**.

22.15 The answer is **A**. Butler and Lewis described systematic life review therapy as "a universal mental process brought about by the realization of approaching disillusion and death which cause the myths of invulnerability and immortality to give way" **(p. 403)**.

22.16 The answer is **A**. Existential psychotherapy is a method of exploration that focuses on the nature of human beings and the person's experience of anxiety **(p. 403)**.

22.17 The answer is **D**. Institutional group psychotherapy can accomplish several goals. Specific goals include halting regression, resocialization, reengagement, problem solving, and information exchange **(p. 404)**.

22.18 The answer is **D**. Group psychotherapy can be completed with elderly persons using issue- or problem-focused support groups. Examples of such groups include retirement adjustment groups, widowhood groups, and groups focused on caregivers of patients with Alzheimer's disease **(p. 406)**.

Psychotherapy **165**

22.19 The answer is **E**. Treatment of the elderly with psychiatric disorders is influenced by developments in scientific knowledge as well as the changing climate of health care. The development of scientific knowledge, the rapid exchange in the health care system, the emphasis on outcomes, and the cost-effectiveness of care are all trends influencing treatment **(p. 396)**.

22.20 The answer is **A**. Chaisson-Stewart identified the problems reported as being deterrents to psychotherapy with the elderly. Age-related rigidity in conducting psychotherapy with the elderly included beliefs that the elders had decreased ability for abstract and new learning, perceptions that defenses and personality characteristics are fixed and immutable, and recognition of the limitations in internal and external resources and choice **(p. 396)**.

22.21 The answer is **B**. Tournier proposed that old age could be a time of a new beginning filled with new interests and activities and spiritual involvement facilitating strategies for growth. Spiritual work resulting in empowerment was emphasized by Thibault as a unique component of old age **(p. 397)**.

22.22 The answer is **E**. Four broad areas of barriers or challenges to psychotherapy have been identified. In the caregiver/patient challenge, psychiatric symptoms are related to medical illness and considered to be untreatable. In the family-related barrier, psychiatric symptoms may be identified as a normal part of aging and minimized. Conflict and family ambivalence and old resentment may mediate against treatment as well. The negative stereotyping of the elderly in a youth-oriented society may influence recommendation for treatment or affect the therapist's countertransference. The health care delivery system and societal issues affect reimbursement **(pp. 397–398)**.

22.23 The answer is **B**. Countertransferences that can occur with a younger therapist treating an older patient may include idealization, unconscious hostility due to anger with the therapist's parents, and avoidance of conflictual material due to deferential respect for the older patient **(p. 398)**. Due to a history of ageism in youth-oriented American society, the younger therapist may have a decreased expectancy of the work that can be accomplished with someone in late life **(p. 397)**. An erotic transference may occur from the older patient to the younger therapist.

22.24 The answer is **B**. Anticipating a shorter life span, older patients frequently show a decreased resistance to change and an increased motivation for therapy **(p. 399)**.

22.25 The answer is **B**. The goals of brief dynamic psychotherapy, a time-limited form of individual psychotherapy, are to achieve symptomatic relief and to enhance self-esteem. The achievement of insight or structural characterological change are not expected **(p. 400)**.

22.26 The answer is **B**. Older women compared with older men were found to show improvement earlier and to maintain their improvement longer from treatment with brief psychodynamic psychotherapy **(p. 400)**.

22.27 The answer is **A**. Gallagher and Thompsen suggested the need for older persons to be socialized to the treatment process. This was required because of the older person's distrust of psychotherapy. Recognizing the age-related perceptual changes (decreased vision and hearing) and the cognitive limitations of the older patient, the therapist should use a variety of modes of learning, including examples specific to the experience of the older patient **(p. 401)**.

22.28 The answer is **E**. The behavioral treatment of depression using cognitive-behavior therapy emphasizes seven components **(p. 401)**. The fourth component addresses learning social skills to enable the older depressed patient to experience pleasant events. Specific skills to be gained include progressive relaxation techniques for stress management, assertiveness training, cognitive skills to decrease or avoid negative thought, social/communication skills, and time management **(p. 401)**.

22.29 The answer is **C**. The primary characteristics of interpersonal therapy include being time limited, being focused, emphasizing current relationships, and being interpersonal rather than intrapsychic **(p. 402)**.

22.30 The answer is **E**. Several factors were identified by Yalom as being limited to change. These factors included instillation of hope, universality, imparting of information, altruism, corrective recapitulation of the primary family group, development of socializing techniques, imitative behavior, interpersonal learning, group cohesiveness, catharsis, and existential factors **(p. 404)**.

22.31 The answer is **E**. Group psychotherapy with elderly patients includes a variety of psychotherapeutic approaches. These include

Psychotherapy

psychodynamic, interpersonal supportive, cognitive-behavior, and expressive approaches **(p. 404)**.

22.32 The answer is **C**. The old assumption that the use of medication interfered with the psychotherapeutic process is acknowledged to be invalid. Combined treatment (psychotherapy and pharmacotherapy) is indicated for patients with more severe depression with associated melancholia or who have only partial responses to either treatment alone. For patients treated with psychotherapy alone with a good response to treatment after 6 weeks or only a practice response after 12 weeks, the addition of medication is indicated **(p. 407)**.

22.33 The answer is **E**. Attention should be paid to the special needs of the elderly. Seating with adequate seat height and arm rests assist the older patient in getting into and out of the chair. Due to decreased visual acuity, the older patient may need lighting two to three times the usual. The use of written material with large print will facilitate communication as well as the assessment process. The use of the older person's surname conveys respect, approval, and affirmation **(p. 408)**.

Chapter 23

Clinical Psychiatry in the Nursing Home

QUESTIONS

Directions: **Select the single best response for each of the following questions.**

23.1 Nursing homes function
- A. To provide long-term care for elderly patients with chronic illness and disability.
- B. To provide rehabilitation for those recovering from acute illness.
- C. To provide convalescent care for those recovering from acute illness.
- D. All of these.
- E. None of these.

23.2 The percentage of Americans age 65 and older residing in more than 20,000 long-term care facilities is
- A. 15%.
- B. 10%.
- C. 5%.
- D. All of these.
- E. None of these.

23.3 Of all nursing home residents, the percentage that are age 65 and older is
- A. 88%.
- B. 78%.
- C. 68%.
- D. All of these.
- E. None of these.

23.4 The mean length of stay in a nursing home was
1. 1.5 years.
2. 2.5 years.
3. 3.5 years.
4. All of these.
5. None of these.

23.5 Among newly admitted nursing home residents, the prevalence rate of psychiatric disorders was reported to be
A. 60%.
B. 80%.
C. 100%.
D. All of these.
E. None of these.

23.6 When followed-up 3.6 years after the diagnosis of depression, the percentage of nursing home residents who had recovered was
A. 17%.
B. 35%.
C. 60%.
D. All of these.
E. None of these.

23.7 Depression among nursing home residents is complicated by
A. The frail condition of the patient.
B. The cooccurrence of depression and medical illness.
C. Frequent occurrence of intercurrent illnesses.
D. All of these.
E. None of these.

23.8 Factors predicting a failure to respond to nortriptyline treatment and suggesting clinically relevant subtype of depression among frail elderly nursing home residents include
A. Level of physical activity.
B. Level of serum total protein.
C. Presence of apraxia.
D. All of these.
E. None of these.

23.9 Potential adverse effects of restraints include
- A. Skin breakdown.
- B. Demoralization.
- C. Disorganized behavior.
- D. All of these.
- E. None of these.

23.10 Historically, 50% of nursing home residents have orders for psychotropic drugs. The most frequently prescribed class of psychoactive medication is
- A. Antidepressants.
- B. Anxiolytics or hypnotics.
- C. Neuroleptics or antipsychotics.
- D. All of these.
- E. None of these.

23.11 Factors contributing to the Omnibus Budget Reconciliation Act (OBRA) of 1987 (Public Law 100-203), written to regulate the operation of nursing facilities and their provision of care, were
- A. The misuse of physical restraints.
- B. The misuse of chemical restraints.
- C. The admission of patients with chronic and severe psychiatric problems to Medicaid-certified nursing homes.
- D. All of these.
- E. None of these.

23.12 Nursing home residents are regularly monitored with the
- A. Mini-Mental State Exam (MMSE).
- B. Geriatric Depression Scale (GDS).
- C. Minimum Data Set (MDS).
- D. All of these.
- E. None of these.

23.13 An *unnecessary drug* is defined as any drug
- A. Used in excessive dose and for excessive duration.
- B. Used with adequate monitoring.
- C. With adequate indications for its use.
- D. All of these.
- E. None of these.

23.14 Subacute patients transferred from acute-care hospitals have primary diagnoses of
   A. Hip fracture.
   B. Stroke.
   C. Cancer.
   D. All of these.
   E. None of these.

Directions: **For each of the statements below, one or more of the answers is correct. Choose**

   A. If 1, 2, and 3 are correct.
   B. If only 1 and 3 are correct.
   C. If only 2 and 4 are correct.
   D. If only 4 is correct.
   E. If all are correct.

23.15 Nursing home residents tend to be very disabled, with over 55%
   1. Requiring assistance in bathing.
   2. Requiring assistance with dressing.
   3. Requiring assistance in toileting and transferring.
   4. Being incontinent.

23.16 Projections about the use of nursing homes indicate that the following percentage of Americans will spend part of their lives in a nursing home
   1. 70%.
   2. 45%.
   3. 50%.
   4. 25%.

23.17 The most common psychiatric disorders identified among nursing home residents are
   1. Dementia.
   2. Depression.
   3. Behavioral disorder in dementia.
   4. Delirium.

Clinical Psychiatry in the Nursing Home 173

23.18 Depression among nursing home residents is associated with
   1. An increase in pain complaints.
   2. An association with biochemical markers of subnutrition.
   3. Increased mortality ranging from 1.6 to 3 (effect size).
   4. A decrease in complaints of anxiety.

23.19 The absence of mental health services in nursing homes or the presence of inadequate services result in
   1. 67% of nursing home residents with psychiatric disorders being misdiagnosed.
   2. Only 5% of the mental health service needs of nursing home residents being met.
   3. The mismanagement of psychiatric problems with physical or chemical restraints.
   4. Mismanagement of "uncomplicated" medical or surgical problems.

23.20 Factors predicting the use of restraints include
   1. Agitation and behavioral problems.
   2. Age and cognitive impairment.
   3. Risk of injury to self (falls) or others (combative behavior).
   4. Physical frailty.

23.21 When the initial first-stage screening identifies serious mental disorder other than dementia, a second-stage psychiatric evaluation is mandated
   1. To ascertain whether the patient has a mental disorder.
   2. To make a specific diagnosis.
   3. To determine whether there is a need for acute psychiatric care that precludes adequate or appropriate treatment in a nursing home.
   4. To prevent the inappropriate admission of patients with severe psychiatric disorder to nursing homes.

23.22 Resident Assessment Protocols (RAP) are designed to help nursing home staff
   1. Recognize common signs and symptom clusters that are indicators of clinically significant problems.
   2. Conduct in-depth evaluations following standardized algorithms.
   3. Determine whether it is necessary to alter the treatment plan.
   4. Identify the need to initiate the mandated physician role in RAP.

174 Study Guide to the Textbook of Geriatric Psychiatry, Second Edition

23.23 RAP problem areas related to mental health behavior include
1. Delirium and cognitive loss/dementia.
2. Psychotropic drug use and physical restraints.
3. Behavioral problems and moved state.
4. Psychosocial well-being.

23.24 The Medicare Prospective Payment System (PPS) has resulted in
1. Decreased length of stay in hospitals.
2. Increased episodes of delirium.
3. Increased transfer of subacute patients to nursing homes.
4. Increased costs for a total episode of care.

ANSWERS

23.1 The answer is **D**. Nursing homes provide long-term care for elderly patients with chronic illness and disability as well as rehabilitative services and convalescent care for those recovering from acute illness **(p. 413)**.

23.2 The answer is **C**. Approximately 5% of Americans age 65 and older reside in more than 20,000 long-term care facilities. This represents some 1.5 million older Americans **(p. 413)**.

23.3 The answer is **A**. The percentage of nursing home residents who are age 65 and older is 88%, with the proportions of individuals living in nursing homes increasing with increasing age **(p. 413)**.

23.4 The answer is **B**. The mean length of stay in a nursing home was 2.5 years, with 67% of residents living in a home for at least 1 year **(p. 413)**.

23.5 The answer is **B**. In a well-controlled study of new admissions to a proprietary chain of nursing homes, 80% of newly admitted patients were found to have psychiatric disorders **(p. 414)**.

23.6 The answer is **A**. Only 17% of nursing home patients with diagnosable depressive disorders had recovered after an average of 3.6 years of follow-up. Depression among nursing home residents tends to be persistent **(p. 415)**.

23.7 The answer is **D**. The treatment of depression among frail elderly nursing home residents with nortriptyline was found to be effective; 58% were rated as much improved on nortriptyline compared with placebo (only 9% much improved). But cooccurring medical illness with depression and the frequent occurrence of intercurrent medical illness complicate the long-term management of these patients **(p. 416)**.

23.8   The answer is **E**. Katz and colleagues (1989b, 1990) showed that measurements of self-care deficits and low levels of serum albumin were intercorrelated, and both predicted a failure to respond to nortriptyline. These authors suggested that these findings might identify a treatment-relevant subtype of depression specific to the nursing home setting **(p. 416)**.

23.9   The answer is **D**. The use of mechanical restraints has potential adverse effects. In addition to skin breakdown, demoralization, and disorganized behavior, the use of restraints increases the risk of falls or other injuries, contributes to functional decline, and produces the physiologic effects of immobilization **(p. 417)**.

23.10 The answer is **C**. When 50% of nursing home residents had orders for psychoactive medications, 20%–40% of orders were for neuroleptic or antipsychotic medication. Some 10%–40% of nursing home residents had an anxiolytic or hypnotic prescribed, and only 5%–10% were taking antidepressants **(p. 417)**.

23.11 The answer is **D**. Federal legislation was developed to address the misuse of physical and chemical restraints in nursing homes by advocacy groups. The U.S. General Accounting Office was concerned that states may have been admitting patients with chronic and severe mental illness to Medicaid-certified nursing homes to shift the costs of care to the federal government. OBRA of 1987 (Public Law 100-203) was the resulting legislation. The Health Care Financing Administration (HFCA) in 1992 issued specific guidelines to assist federal and state surveyors in interpreting the legislation **(p. 418)**.

23.12 The answer is **C**. The MDS was identified by the HCFA guidelines as the instrument to provide a comprehensive assessment of nursing home residents. Areas of assessment relevant to mental illness and behavior include mood, cognition, communication, functional status, medication, and other treatments. Responses to the MDS suggest that there may need to be a reassessment of the patient's clinical status and treatment plan. These findings trigger the RAP **(p. 418)**.

23.13 The answer is **A**. The HCFA defined an *unnecessary drug* as any drug used in excessive dose and for excessive duration. Other criteria included any drug used without adequate monitoring, any drug used without any adequate indication for its use, any drug continued in the presence of adverse consequences that indicate it should be reduced or discontinued, or any combination of these reasons **(p. 419)**.

23.14 The answer is **D**. Subacute patients transferred to nursing homes from acute-care hospitals have primary diagnoses of hip fracture, stroke, and cancer. They differ from the long-term care patients in being younger, more likely to be admitted from an acute-care hospital, and less likely to have irreversible cognitive impairment or incontinence **(p. 420)**.

23.15 The answer is **E**. The extent of disability of nursing home residents is shown by the following statistics: 91% of all residents require assistance in bathing, 78% need help with dressing, 63% need assistance in both toileting and transferring, 55% are incontinent, and 40% require help with eating. Only 8% of nursing home residents were found to be independent in all activities of daily living **(p. 413)**.

23.16 The answer is **D**. Projection by Campion et al. (1983) indicates that 25% of Americans will spend part of their lives in a nursing home. By 2020, that figure is projected to triple **(p. 413)**.

23.17 The answer is **E**. Among nursing home residents, some 50%–75% have a diagnosis of dementia. Of these patients, 50%–60% have primary degenerative dementia of the Alzheimer's type, and 25%–30% have multiinfarct dementia. Delirium and behavioral disturbances may complicate dementia. The second most common psychiatric disorder among nursing home residents is depression **(pp. 414–415)**. The prevalence rates of depression in U.S. nursing homes range from 15% to 50% **(p. 415)**.

23.18 The answer is **A**. Depression among nursing home residents is associated with increased morbidity, increased complaints of pain, and an association with biochemical markers of subnutrition and mortality. Mortality among depressed nursing home residents is increased with effect sizes of 1.6–3 **(p. 415)**.

23.19 The answer is **A**. Nursing homes were designed to provide treatment for "uncomplicated" medical and surgical cases. With inadequate mental health services, 67% of nursing home residents with psychiatric disorders are misdiagnosed, and only 5% of the mental health service needs of nursing home residents are being met. The mismanagement of psychiatric problems with physical and chemical restraints is a consequence of the absence of psychiatric services resulting in neglect of diagnosis and inappropriate treatment **(p. 416)**.

Clinical Psychiatry in the Nursing Home   177

23.20   The answer is **E**. In addition to agitation and behavioral problems, mechanical restraints are used on nursing home residents who have the following factors: age, cognitive impairment, risk of injury to self (for example, falls) or to others (for example, combative behavior), physical frailty, the presence of monitoring or treatment devices, and the need to promote body alignment **(p. 417)**.

23.21   The answer is **E**. The Preadmission Screening and Annual Resident Review (PASARR) is a two-stage process. It is a required assessment of every resident before admission to any nursing home. When the first-stage (initial) screening identifies a serious mental illness other than dementia, a second-stage evaluation is completed by a psychiatrist. This required psychiatric evaluation determines whether the patient has a mental illness, makes a specific psychiatric diagnosis, and determines whether there is a need for acute psychiatric care that precludes adequate or appropriate treatment in a nursing home. The purpose of this two-stage preadmission screening is to prevent inappropriate admission of patients with severe psychiatric disorders to nursing homes and to help ensure that patients with disabilities due to treatable psychiatric disorders (e.g., depression) are not placed in long-term care facilities before they receive adequate psychiatric treatment **(p. 418)**.

23.22   The answer is **A**. Physicians have no mandated role in the RAPs. The RAPs are designed to help nursing home staff recognize common sign and symptom clusters that are indicators of clinically significant problems, to conduct in-depth evaluations following standardized algorithms, and to determine whether it is necessary to alter the treatment plan **(p. 418)**.

23.23   The answer is **E**. The problem areas related to mental health and behavior of the RAP include delirium, cognitive loss/dementia, psychosocial well-being, mood state, behavior problems, psychotropic drug use, and physical restraints **(p. 418)**.

23.24   The answer is **B**. The PPS established payment for acute-care hospitals based on diagnosis-related groups rather than length of stay. Hospitals became more concerned with limiting the length of stay in the hospital to decrease costs and have increasingly discharged subacute patients to nursing homes as "step-down" facilities that provide subacute medical treatment, convalescent care, and rehabilitation services. The transfer of subacute hospital patients to nursing homes has resulted in 33% of nursing home admissions being such subacute patients **(p. 420)**.

CHAPTER 24

The Continuum of Care

Movement Toward the Community

QUESTIONS

Directions: **Select the single best response for each of the following questions.**

24.1 American health care has focused on
   A. Preventive medicine.
   B. Community-based care.
   C. Teams of professionals and paraprofessionals.
   D. All of these.
   E. None of these.

24.2 Nursing homes in the United States are viewed as hospitals that are
   A. Second rate.
   B. Understaffed.
   C. Underfunded.
   D. All of these.
   E. None of these.

24.3 The movement of the chronically mentally ill from mental hospitals to long-term care facilities was facilitated by
   A. Medicare.
   B. Medicaid.
   C. Social Security.
   D. All of these.
   E. None of these.

24.4 A major factor in the transformation of the health care system from hospital-based care to community-based care will be
   A. Public opinion.
   B. Political feasibility.
   C. Financial resources.
   D. All of these.
   E. None of these.

24.5 Based on the Channeling Project data and smaller studies, the most likely way to reduce or moderate total system cost is to
   A. Screen older persons to determine the care needed.
   B. Assign each elder needing care to a community site.
   C. Place all elderly in a system with a capped organizational budget.
   D. All of these.
   E. None of these.

24.6 The health maintenance organization (HMO) concept is identified as responding to the needs of older persons for comprehensive care. The cost-effectiveness obtained by HMOs is due to
   A. A restriction to access to care.
   B. An emphasis on prevention.
   C. A reduction of institutionalization.
   D. All of these.
   E. None of these.

24.7 The Scottish health care model studied in Glasgow had
   A. A primary care health center as its focal point.
   B. A staff including general practioners, visiting nurses, and social workers.
   C. Access to a continuum of alternative care settings.
   D. All of these.
   E. None of these.

Directions: **For each of the statements below, one or more of the answers is correct. Choose**

   A. If 1, 2, and 3 are correct.
   B. If only 1 and 3 are correct.
   C. If only 2 and 4 are correct.
   D. If only 4 is correct.
   E. If all are correct.

The Continuum of Care

24.8 Data on older Americans reveal that 60% have no significant impairment in
   1. Social support network.
   2. Economic security.
   3. Physical health and mental health.
   4. The capacity to perform basic physical activities of daily living.

24.9 Approximately 12%–15% of older persons in the community
   1. Are seriously impaired.
   2. Are placed in a nursing home.
   3. Receive services provided by family and friends.
   4. Receive Medicare home health aides.

24.10 The "consequences of modernization" thesis suggests that the dependent old will be vulnerable to
   1. Isolation.
   2. Social irrelevance.
   3. Neglect.
   4. Poverty.

24.11 The high degree of specialization in contemporary health care in the United States
   1. Results in acute problems of fragmentation.
   2. Requires organizational coordination.
   3. Results in gaps in coverage.
   4. Excludes community and home care.

24.12 The National Long-Term Care Demonstration Project, known as the Channeling Project, found
   1. The costs of expanded case management and community services were not offset by reductions in nursing home and other costs.
   2. The demonstration increased client and informal caregiver confidence and life satisfaction.
   3. No significant affect in client function or risk of mortality.
   4. The channeling interventions did not reduce the relatively heavy use of physicians and medical services.

24.13 Although lower total system costs for long-term care were not achieved, health status effects across all studies found
1. An improvement in life satisfaction for both services.
2. A decrease in mortality.
3. A reduction in unmet needs.
4. A decrease in hospital costs.

24.14 Behavioral and lifestyle changes that would decrease the risk of mortality and morbidity include
1. Ceasing smoking.
2. Ceasing overeating.
3. Increasing physical activity.
4. Using seat belts.

24.15 The unconditional autonomy and medical monopoly of health care in the United States have been challenged with
1. Due process.
2. Medical licensure.
3. Restraint of trade.
4. Quality control.

ANSWERS

24.1 The answer is **E**. The American health care system focuses on acute hospital care dependent on high technology and controlled by highly specialized personnel centralized in or near hospitals **(p. 436)**.

24.2 The answer is **D**. Long-stay institutions have a negative image in the United States. Nursing homes are viewed as being second-rate, understaffed, and underfunded hospitals **(p. 436)**.

24.3 The answer is **B**. The reimbursement structure of Medicaid is an important factor in the transfer of patients from mental hospitals to nursing homes **(p. 437)**.

24.4 The answer is **B**. Although the HMO model of care has been identified as the best model for the provision of assessment, health care, sick care, and preventive maintenance, the national adoption of this model will be influenced by its political feasibility and its ability to please those who have the authority to decide and to allocate resources **(p. 434)**.

The Continuum of Care 183

24.5 The answer is **C**. The Channeling Project used screening and referred older persons to community sites without a reduction in costs in nursing home and other costs. Based on the Channeling Project data and other smaller studies, the reduction of total system cost was believed to be accomplished best by a capped organizational budget covering inpatient, outpatient, and community care service **(p. 446)**.

24.6 The answer is **C**. The cost-effectiveness of HMOs has been established and attributed to a reduction of institutionalization not to a restriction of access to care. The HMO model meets the needs of older persons for comprehensive care **(p. 453)**.

24.7 The answer is **D**. The Scottish Home and Health Service, the Scottish health care model, has a long tradition of integrating medical and social services and is, by definition, a comprehensive, prepaid care system. Its focal point is a primary care health center staffed by general practioners, visiting nurses, and social workers trained as a team. This multidisciplinary team has access to an extensive continuum of alternative care settings, including in-home services, day care, day hospitals, sheltered housing, and inpatient hospital services, with both general and specialized hospital wards including geriatric psychiatry **(p. 454)**.

24.8 The answer is **E**. Although 80% of older adults have at least one chronic condition, 60% of older persons are not significantly impaired in five important dimensions of functioning. These five dimensions include social support network, economic security, physical health, mental health, and capacity for performing basic physical and management activities of daily living **(p. 440)**.

24.9 The answer is **B**. Although 12%–15% of community-resident elderly have serious impairment, 80% of these older persons receive services provided by family and friends **(p. 440)**.

24.10 The answer is **A**. The hypotheses of the "consequences of modernization" thesis is that the price of industrialization, urbanization, and rapid social change will be the weakening of familial and community ties. Dependent elderly would become vulnerable to isolation, social irrelevance, and neglect. The high divorce rate, increase in single parent families, and use of experts to resolve personal and family problems reflect a change in family structure and function in recent decades **(p. 440)**.

24.11 The answer is **A**. A high degree of specialization characterizes contemporary health care in the United States. This specialization includes community and home care. The absence of limits to the permutations and combinations of specialized people, activities, and locals produces acute problems of fragmentation requiring organizational coordination and tends to have gaps in coverage **(pp. 441, 449)**.

24.12 The answer is **E**. The National Long-Term Care Demonstration Project (Channeling Project) was to assess the effects of comprehensive case management of community care on cost containment in long-term care without sacrificing quality of care for the needy impaired elderly. The study results found increased client and informal caregiver confidence and life satisfaction, but costs were not reduced, mortality was not reduced, informal care was unaffected by the demonstration project, and the subpopulation at highest risk was not identified **(p. 445)**.

24.13 The answer is **B**. Data across all studies showed no reduction in total system costs for long-term care with the introduction of home and community-care services. Health status effects consistently reported across studies were 1) improvements in life satisfaction for persons receiving home- or community-care services and their caregivers and 2) a reduction of unmet needs **(p. 447)**.

24.14 The answer is **E**. Cigarette smoking, overeating, physical inactivity, and nonuse of seat belts are all modifiable behaviors and lifestyle patterns that increase morbidity and mortality. Changing these patterns would decrease mortality and morbidity. Social controls intended to modify risky behavior or noxious environmental factors are interpreted as infringements on personal freedom **(p. 451)**.

24.15 The answer is **E**. Beginning in the 14th century, laws regulating professional malpractice have evolved. The increasing public challenge of unconditional professional autonomy and a medical monopoly of health care resources is reflected in laws dealing with due process, licensure, restraint of trade, and quality control **(p. 452)**.